"Cutting-edge information from two leading researchers . . . excellent."

—*Library Journal*

"The most comprehensive and readable reference available today for diagnosis, treatment, and delaying the onset of Alzheimer's disease and related disorders . . . a medical text on dementia for the lay reader."

—Charles Parker, D.O.,
psychopharmacologist, psychiatrist, and author of *Deep Recovery*

"*Preventing Alzheimer's* is practical, useful, and up-to-date. How could anyone not want to read this book? Given how devastating Alzheimer's is, we all should do whatever we can to stave it off or prevent it altogether. This is the best guide I know of on how to do that."

—Edward Hallowell, M.D.,
author of *The Childhood Roots of Adult Happiness*
and *Driven to Distraction*

"I heartily recommend this book to all. Alzheimer's disease is not an incurable illness, but one for which we have not yet found the cure. There is much that can be done now to reduce your risk."

—William H. Frey II, Ph.D.,
director, Alzheimer's Research Center

"This superb book is both clear and clinically sound, breathtakingly comprehensive and simply practical. I loved the integration of advice on supplements and nutraceuticals with up-to-the-minute medical information. *Preventing Alzheimer's* will be on my desk for my own use, and I will be recommending it to many patients."

—Thomas M. Brod, M.D.,
assistant clinical professor of psychiatry, UCLA School of Medicine

"A must-read for those at risk for memory problems. An ounce of prevention is worth a pound of cure."

—Mark Kosins, M.D.,
assistant clinical professor of psychiatry and human behavior,
University of California, Irvine

continued . . .

D0197232

"It is now inconceivable that our society should continue to face the likelihood of dementia as unavoidable. Patients and society alike can benefit from the concepts reported in this book."

—Steven Richard Devore Best, M.D.,
director, The Neuroscience Center, LLC

"A fresh and demystifying look at a topic that has for years kindled fear in the soul of our generation. It will forever change our view of aging and the way we manage and maintain our faculties."

—Scott L. Fairchild, Psy.D.,
president, Baytree Behavioral Health,
and director, Disaster Mental Health Services Support Team,
Kennedy Space Center, NASA

"Relevant and easily understandable information which unites health care providers and the public as well-informed partners in dealing with the existence of Alzheimer's disease."

—Dr. Anthony Clark, medical director,
Cook County Hospital Westside Ambulatory Care Clinic

"A book of hope and encouragement. If you have one relative with dementia or Alzheimer's, buy this book. I am going to be recommending this book to each patient I see [and] family member, and am already following the prevention protocols for myself. Never before have I read a book that is so practical and will move you to action."

—Earl R. Henslin, Psy.D., B.C.E.T.S.,
board-certified expert in Traumatic Stress

"A fresh new approach to assessing and treating Alzheimer's disease. The book inspires the reader with valuable explanations of the various Alzheimer's-type illnesses, and is a must for anyone who seeks answers in the understanding and dealing with those suffering from progressive memory loss."

—Matthew S. Stubblefield, M.D.,
general child and adult psychiatry

continued . . .

"Anyone who suspects that he or she might be developing the disorder, or whose spouse or adult children might worry about the possibility, should get this book. It is very well written, and extremely helpful and hopeful. I am happy to recommend it."

—R. George Christie, M.D., F.R.C.P,
child psychiatrist

"A very encouraging and wonderfully practical guide to this condition. . . . Their 'steps to prevention' section motivated me to improve upon the preventative measures that I have already been using."

—J. Michael Uszler, M.D.,
Santa Monica Imaging and Therapy Associates

"*Preventing Alzheimer's* translates the latest research into useful information. With understanding comes the possibility of significantly reducing the incidence, and delaying the onset of this great thief of our senior citizens' mental life."

—Timmen L. Cermack, M.D.,
author of *Marijuana: What's a Parent to Believe?*

"[E]xplores not only accepted medical treatment, but also looks at contributions from alternative medicine, and attempts to provide a balanced perspective on somewhat controversial therapies. I highly recommend this text to anyone, physician or layman, interested in increasing his understanding of this tragically common disease."

—Philip Cohen, M.D., F.R.C.P. (C.), A.B.N.M.,
clinical associate professor, Radiology;
division head, Nuclear Medicine, University of British Columbia

"Both easy to read and vastly informative . . . offers practical, useful approaches to identifying and treating Alzheimer's disease."

—William C. Klindt, M.D.,
diplomate, American Board of Psychiatry and Neurology;
director, Silicon Valley Brain SPECT Imaging

continued . . .

"A thorough, up-to-date, well-constructed, informative exploration of what we know about the clinical features, diagnosis, and current research and applied efforts to prevent Alzheimer's and other dementias, which are reviewed and lucidly described in this book. *Preventing Alzheimer's* provides a real service to the public at large, who will find in it many answers to their questions as well as the factual grounding that will enable them to evaluate new research as it emerges over the next decade. The authors should be congratulated for their effort."

—Barton J. Blinder, M.D., Ph.D.
Clinical Professor, Department of Psychiatry and Human Behavior, College of Medicine, University of California, Irvine

Most Perigee Books are available at special quantity discounts for bulk purchases for sales promotions, premiums, fund-raising, or educational use. Special books, or book excerpts, can also be created to fit specific needs.

For details, write: Special Markets, The Berkley Publishing Group, 375 Hudson Street, New York, New York 10014.

OTHER BOOKS BY DANIEL G. AMEN, M.D.

Healing Anxiety and Depression with Lisa C. Routh, M.D.

Healing the Hardware of the Soul

Healing ADD

Change Your Brain, Change Your Life

New Skills for Frazzled Parents

Would You Give Two Minutes a Day for a Lifetime of Love?

Coaching Yourself to Success

Firestorms in the Brain: An Inside Look at Violence

Secrets of Successful Students

ADD and Relationships

A Teenager's Guide to ADD

A Sibling's Guide to ADD

A Teacher's Guide to ADD

OTHER BOOKS BY WILLIAM RODMAN SHANKLE, M.S., M.D.

The Developing Human Brain

Computational Neuroanatomy

William Rodman Shankle, M.S., M.D., and
Daniel G. Amen, M.D.

Preventing Alzheimer's

Ways to Help Prevent,

Delay, Detect,

and Even Halt

Alzheimer's Disease

and Other Forms of

Memory Loss

A Perigee Book

THE BERKLEY PUBLISHING GROUP
Published by the Penguin Group
Penguin Group (USA) Inc.
375 Hudson Street, New York, New York 10014, USA
Penguin Group (Canada), 10 Alcorn Avenue, Toronto, Ontario M4V 3B2, Canada
(a division of Pearson Penguin Canada Inc.)
Penguin Books Ltd., 80 Strand, London WC2R 0RL, England
Penguin Ireland, 25 St. Stephen's Green, Dublin 2, Ireland (a division of Penguin Books Ltd.)
Penguin Group (Australia), 250 Camberwell Road, Camberwell, Victoria 3124, Australia
(a division of Pearson Australia Group Pty. Ltd.)
Penguin Books India Pvt. Ltd., 11 Community Centre, Panchsheel Park, New Delhi–110 017, India
Penguin Group (NZ), Cnr Airborne and Rosedale Roads, Albany, Auckland 1310, New Zealand
(a division of Pearson New Zealand Ltd.)
Penguin Books (South Africa) (Pty.) Ltd., 24 Sturdee Avenue, Rosebank, Johannesburg 2196, South Africa
Penguin Books Ltd., Registered Offices: 80 Strand, London WC2R 0RL, England

Copyright © 2004 by William Rodman Shankle, M.S., M.D., and Daniel G. Amen, M.D.
Cover design © by Jae Song

Every effort has been made to ensure that the information contained in this book is complete and accurate. However, neither the publisher nor the authors are engaged in rendering professional advice or services to the individual reader. The ideas, procedures, and suggestions contained in this book are not intended as a substitute for consulting with your physician. All matters regarding your health require medical supervision. Neither the authors nor the publisher shall be liable or responsible for any loss or damage allegedly arising from any information or suggestion in this book. The opinions expressed in this book represent the personal views of the authors and not of the publisher. While the authors have made every effort to provide accurate telephone numbers and Internet addresses at the time of publication, neither the publisher nor the authors assume any responsibility for errors, or for changes that occur after publication.

All rights reserved. This book, or parts thereof, may not be reproduced, scanned, or distributed in any printed or electronic form without permission. Please do not participate in or encourage piracy of copyrighted materials in violation of the author's rights. Purchase only authorized editions.

PRINTING HISTORY
Perigee trade paperback edition / June 2005

PERIGEE is a registered trademark of Penguin Group (USA) Inc.
The "P" design is a trademark belonging to Penguin Group (USA) Inc.

ISBN 0-399-53160-2

The Library of Congress has cataloged the G. P. Putnam's Sons hardcover as follows

Shankle, William Rodman.
    Preventing Alzheimer's : ways to help prevent, detect, diagnose, treat, and even halt Alzheimer's disease and other causes of memory loss / William Rodman Shankle, Daniel G. Amen.
        p. cm.
    Includes bibliographical references and index.
    ISBN 0-399-15155-9
    1. Alzheimer's disease—Prevention.   I. Amen, Daniel G.   II. Title
RC523.S525   2004   2003066431
616.8'3105—dc22

PRINTED IN THE UNITED STATES OF AMERICA

10   9   8   7   6   5

Contents

By Leeza Gibbons, Founder,
The Leeza Gibbons Memory Foundation

Foreword

If you've picked up this book, you're probably scared. Or if not afraid, at least interested in what causes Alzheimer's disease and learning whether you are at risk.

The reality is that we're all at risk of having this "terrorist-like thief" randomly break into our brains and begin to rewrite our life stories. As Baby Boomers beginning to face our mortality, Alzheimer's is the unwelcome stranger that reminds us of our vulnerability.

The good news is that we don't have to be defenseless.

My grandmother lost her life because of Alzheimer's disease. We lose a little more of my mom everyday. Before Mom was fully trapped behind the fog, she asked me to promise that I would tell her story and use it to educate and inspire. I am, but doing so often brings more questions than answers. She looked into the face of her mother at my Granny's funeral knowing what her fate would be. I looked at Mom and wondered . . . What about my children, and what about me? Am I next in line to have my memories stolen?

When my three children ask me if I will get "it" I tell them—truthfully— that I don't know.

Thanks to Drs. William Rodman Shankle and Daniel Amen, what I do know is that perhaps I can effectively manage my risk of getting the disease, and you can, too. Whether or not you have a history of Alzheimer's or dementia in your family, your goal is to keep your brain strong and healthy.

This book will give you all the information you need that may prevent or delay the effects of Alzheimer's from invading your life and stealing from you the memories that are so precious.

It's easy to get overwhelmed and confused by all the information and misinformation out there. Being frustrated and feeling hopeless are by-products for most of us who have tried to unravel the mystery of this disease. This book will explain the kinds of protection you are likely to get from particular supplements or diet changes. It provides specific information about what to take, along with when and how much. It's reassuring and easy to follow. It actually asks *and answers* the questions we hear so often about this disease—and does so in a succinct, thorough way.

We all know that the "age wave" is about to crash in our culture and yet we are not at all ready. Even in the wake of President Ronald Reagan's death, there is still so much shame and stigma surrounding memory disorders that many families try to compensate and deny until they are bankrupt—financially, spiritually, and emotionally. Alzheimer's is a disease that depletes and depletes, and it is never satisfied with the diagnosed individual . . . it wants the entire family.

It's for this reason I created the Leeza Gibbons Memory Foundation. Our family was numb and paralyzed with fear when Mom was diagnosed. It was almost impossible to find the help and support we needed. Answers were scarce.

We wanted to help families connect the dots in their communities. We wanted to offer comfort and care while working toward a cure, and so we created Leeza's Place—intimate, safe, community resource centers for those newly diagnosed with any memory disorder, and their caregivers. It offers a place where families in distress can get education, empowerment, and energy as they prepare for the journey ahead.

I am so amazed to see my mother's love and her spirit used in such a powerful way. She asked me to tell her story and make it count. Every time we help another family at Leeza's Place, that's just what we are doing. Mom is in the final stages of the disease now, but when I see her, I always tell her that I am doing my best to fulfill the promise I made to her.

At Leeza's Place, our mantra is early diagnosis. We believe in memory screenings to get a baseline reading, against which any decline can be measured. We believe in educating our guests about the latest in alternative treatments to complement traditional approaches. We believe in being proactive against this frightening force. We believe in support for both the recently diagnosed and those who care for them.

That's why I am so impressed with Drs. Shankle and Amen and their work. They are well-respected scientists whose work is world renowned, but I also know them as kind, compassionate men who not only focus on how to tackle this disease, but on connecting with families who arrive in their offices with their breath knocked out of them, looking for a miracle. These two doctors will never try to talk anyone out of expecting a good outcome . . . they have seen it happen too many times. They have been the guiding forces toward success stories that may offer real hope against a dark landscape of despair.

When I was a little girl, my mother used to rub my back at bedtime and sing me to sleep. A favorite of hers was the Doris Day classic, "Que Sera, Sera." I remember being comforted by her soothing voice, but I never liked those lyrics, and I still don't believe in what they say. "*Que sera, sera—* whatever will be, will be. The future's not ours to see—*que sera, sera.*"

The words always made me feel so powerless. It's true, of course—the future is *not* ours to see—but it's not a matter of "whatever will be, will be" . . . it's a matter of whatever we can do that might change it—*that's* what the future will be!

You are perhaps doing nothing short of changing the course of your future, and possibly someone else's, by reading this book. Can you think of anything more powerful or important? It's a popular notion that we must gracefully surrender the things of youth. Yes, we will lose our firm muscles and unlined skin, but memories should be ours for keeps. They are what resonate at the end of a life, sweetened over time.

We must do what we can to bolt the door to our minds so that our treasured recollections of those we love, where we went, and what we felt will be kept forever as a sort of "soul print" of our time here on earth. This book suggests options that might have the potential to lock out Alzheimer's disease in order to do just that.

Thank you to Drs. Daniel Amen and William Rodman Shankle for recognizing what so many of us have been looking for, and for providing it to us in this book.

Take a deep breath and read on.

Preventing Alzheimer's

chapter 1

The Power of
"Prevention Through Delay"

Alzheimer's disease (AD) begins an average of 30 years before the first symptoms. The accumulation of beta amyloid plaques in the brain, a major mechanism thought to cause AD, begins as early as 30 years old. It is never too early to start preventing this devastating disease. The good news is that through prevention strategies you may be able to delay the onset of AD long enough so that you will never have symptoms.

One out of every two families in the United States has a member with Alzheimer's disease. It affects approximately five million people in our country, and the chance of developing AD doubles every five years after the age of 65. By age 85, there is a 50 percent chance you will develop AD. The average cost to the family with a member with AD is $200,000–$400,000 over the average eight- to ten-year course of the illness. The average cost to the United States is estimated to be $100 billion annually. Beyond the financial cost, and potentially more devastating, is the severe psychological and social pain many families suffer. Losing a loved one's mind, even though they seem to have a healthy body, coupled with the chronic stress of having to caretake an adult every minute, can exact a heavy toll.

As we write this book, we are both in our late forties and both have family members who suffer from serious memory problems. In addition, we have both dealt with Alzheimer's disease and related disorders (ADRD) professionally for more than 20 years.

Dr. Shankle has seen more than 7,000 patients with ADRD. Several years ago, at an Alzheimer's Association gala to honor Maureen Reagan that he attended, the executive director said, "Alzheimer's disease not only robs people of their minds and humanity, it also destroys their families." Dr. Shankle did not realize how soon this prophecy would come to pass in his own family.

Dr. Amen recently suffered the loss of a good friend from a form of dementia called frontal temporal lobe dementia, which robbed this woman of her very personality. Cathy was a vibrant woman who in two years went from being the center of her family's world to someone no one knew; from being energetic and involved to sitting alone for hours with no interest in going out or being with the people she loved. Ultimately, she had to go to a long-term-care facility, where she eventually died. In addition, Dr. Amen's uncle has been diagnosed with dementia, probably due to a past head injury and severe sleep apnea. Dr. Amen struggled to help his own family deal with many of the common problems families face when dealing with a loved one who has dementia.

It is our sincere hope that you will never have to face the devastating diagnosis of Alzheimer's disease or a related disorder. It is perhaps the most feared illness in the world today. There is much you can do to prevent it, if you start early. This book will give you and your family practical information about preventing and delaying the onset and progression of ADRD. This knowledge can literally help one keep one's mind sharp for as long as possible, stay independent, avoid becoming a burden to one's family, and stay out of a nursing home.

Despite how awful Alzheimer's can be, many people remain in denial because they don't believe they can do anything about it and don't know that early awareness can lead to positive action. Contrary to popular belief, with current medical and scientific knowledge, the onset and progression of ADRD can be delayed by an average of six years. That delay can reduce by half the total number of people who develop the symptoms of ADRD. This means that you may never develop the symptoms of ADRD during your lifetime. These remarkable medical and scientific advances in ADRD research allow you to benefit from the concept of *prevention through delay*, which means that if you can delay the onset and progression of the symptoms of a disease long enough, you will live out your natural life without suffering from that disease.

The concept of *prevention through delay* is very useful in preventing the disability that occurs with many diseases of aging. Once we hit age 40, we have fulfilled our evolutionary purpose of perpetuating the species. After that, from a biologic perspective, we are on our own. The daily repair to the cells of the brain and body can no longer keep up with the daily damage, and our functioning begins to decline. What we do to protect ourselves from the variety of mechanisms that cause this damage to our cells, tissues, and organs allows us to prevent diseases of aging by delaying their onset and progression.

What Can You Do?

In this book we offer a new research- and brain-based program to help people prevent ADRD, recognize it early, and delay its ravaging effects as long as possible. In addition, this book emphasizes the genetic nature of the illness; if one family member is shown to be at risk, other family members can get screened early and become involved in an active prevention program. This book also offers readers a new approach to keeping the mind healthy through supplements, as well as physical and intellectual exercise. By following the program outlined in this book, readers will be able to employ early-detection screening tools and early-intervention strategies to dramatically delay the onset and progression of ADRD.

By utilizing the information in this book, readers will be able to:

- Identify their own personal risk for ADRD
- Identify the risk to their loved ones
- Use healthy brain strategies to help prevent the onset of ADRD
- Employ early treatment strategies at the earliest signs of ADRD to delay or even halt the progression of the illness
- Understand appropriate assessment for ADRD
- Provide information and support for families suffering with one or more forms of dementia

The book is illustrated with many SPECT (single photon emission computed tomography) images, a revolutionary brain imaging method that allows physicians and patients to see how an individual's brain works. SPECT is a nuclear medicine technique that looks at brain blood flow and activity patterns. The SPECT images allow for better and earlier diagnosis, as they more sensitively track the course of the condition as well as the effects of treatment. The images visually help readers understand ADRD and clearly show how proper treatment can optimize brain function.

New Information Leads to New Prevention and Treatment Strategies

As knowledge about dementia and aging accumulate, certain patterns are becoming clear. Unlike most diseases of the young, diseases of aging involve multiple factors. When damage exceeds the brain's ability to repair itself, the first symptoms begin. For example, we now know that memory loss begins in Alzheimer's disease when the entorhinal cortex, an area of brain involved in building new memories, loses neurons faster than they are being replaced.

It was previously thought that we have all of the brain cells we will ever have at birth. In the 1990s, together with his colleagues, Dr. Shankle discovered that the human brain can generate new nerve cells or neurons after birth (1, 2). Subsequent discoveries by Fred Gage and others demonstrated that the human and primate brains continue to make neurons in the cerebral cortex throughout the life span (3). The number of neurons in each brain area tends to stay relatively constant; it was discovered that the number of new neurons produced matches the number of neurons lost in each area. However, when the production of new neurons in a brain region does not keep up with the number of neurons that are dying or being removed, then the functioning of that brain region begins to decline. In the case of Alzheimer's disease, short-term memory begins to fail when the number of neurons in the entorhinal cortex is reduced by about one-third.

Understanding the causes of brain cell loss is relevant to understanding how to effectively prevent diseases of aging in the brain. In Alzheimer's disease, there are a number of ways brain cells die.

1. *Formation of chemicals called free radicals*, which kill brain cells. A lack of antioxidants that protect the brain from free radical formation may be partially to blame.
2. *Too much of a neurotransmitter called glutamate* is released in large quantities when the brain is damaged. Excessive amounts of glutamate further damages brain cells.
3. *An accumulation of a substance called beta amyloid* disrupts brain cell pathways and short-circuits the brain.
4. *Beta amyloid triggers a strong inflammatory response*, which further damages the brain.
5. *A protein called tau*, which forms the backbone of nerve cells in the brain, becomes twisted and interrupts nerve cell function. Eventually, the twisted tau proteins completely block nerve cell function, and the cell dies. It is then called a neurofibrillary tangle.

In the case of Alzheimer's disease, there are now objective data to show that:

1. Certain antioxidants, including vitamin E (4, 5) ginkgo biloba (6, 7), and possibly alpha lipoic acid (8), have significant disease-delaying effects.
2. Agents that prevent overstimulation by the neurotransmitter glutamate have significant benefits in delaying the disease (9).
3. Exelon (10), Reminyl, and Aricept—agents that enhance the neurotransmitter acetylcholine, a key brain substance involved with mem-

ory—help delay AD for six months to three or more years. The earlier treatment starts, the more the disease progression is delayed.

4. Nine out of ten population-based studies have shown that low doses (e.g., 200 to 400 mg of ibuprofen) of nonsteroidal anti-inflammatory agents taken for two or more years in persons under 80 years old reduce the chance of developing AD by about 50 percent (11,12,13,14).
5. To date, the only nonsteroidal agents that block the production of beta amyloid—a key component of AD pathology—are ibuprofen (Motrin, Advil), sulindac, and indomethacin (Indocin).
6. Most studies of aspirin and AD risk show that low-dose aspirin (175 mg or less) reduces the chance of developing AD by 33 to 50 percent.
7. Structured activity programs delays disease progression and institutionalization (15, 16).
8. Regular exercise probably delays disease progression (17).

Unfortunately, the body's production of the antioxidants that protect cells from damage decline with age. Different antioxidants such as vitamin E, vitamin C, coenzyme Q10, and ginkgo biloba protect different parts of the cell. No one antioxidant will "do it all."

Exercise, which also decreases with age for many, has many helpful effects on the brain. It increases the levels of nerve growth factors in the brain, which has been seen in young animals to stimulate new brain cell formation and help strengthen connections between brain cells (the synapses). Exercise also improves the strength of the heart muscle so that the deep areas of the brain receive better blood flow. It is these deep areas of the brain that are the most susceptible to reduced blood flow and cellular damage as we age. The well-designed Canadian Study of Health and Aging, which followed 4,615 cognitively normal Canadians over 65 years old for five years, found that regular physical exercise reduced dementia risk by 50 percent (18).

Certain over-the-counter medications, such as anti-inflammatory agents—including aspirin, ibuprofen, naproxen, and other "arthritis" drugs—reduce the risk of developing Alzheimer's disease by as much as 55 percent (11). However, the benefits do not appear to be related to the anti-inflammatory effect because low doses are just as effective as high doses. Some, but not all of these compounds block the production of beta amyloid. One study has shown that memory loss and other cognitive impairment are delayed by an average of three and a half years in people under 80 years old who take anti-inflammatory medication on a regular basis for at least two years (19).

We will discuss other factors, including hypertension, stress, alcohol, tobacco, and so on, that one can modify in preventing Alzheimer's disease, but the big picture should be clear. We are promoting an approach to living that emphasizes balance. We live in a fast-paced, fast-food society that leaves many lives out of balance. If we wish to age in a healthy way, we must optimize or alter our current and future lifestyle behaviors. Such an approach can minimize the multitude of factors that add up to damaged brain tissue that can ultimately become dementia.

One of the fundamental problems of prevention is in knowing what combination of treatments is right for each individual. We will present an approach that is cost-effective by allowing you to tailor prevention strategies to your risks.

Stacey ❖ Early Diagnosis

Stacey was a 54-year-old schoolteacher who was brought in by her husband for evaluation. Stacey had been having trouble teaching her usual classes, had angry outbursts for seemingly trivial problems, and was starting to alienate her children and colleagues. She also forgot meetings with her other teachers, was late paying bills (very unlike her), and got lost twice in a town she had lived in for 32 years. She attributed these problems to a lifelong history of anxiety combined with stress due to the loss of her father, who had recently died of Alzheimer's disease. Her family doctor agreed that stress was the cause of her problems. Stacey's husband, John, and her daughter, Jacqueline, were more concerned about her behavior than she was. John's biggest fear was that his wife had early AD, a common and serious cause of senility that has strong genetic underpinnings. Jacqueline's biggest fear was that she was going to develop AD in the future.

Stacey was evaluated with a computerized screening battery and a

Figures 1.1-2. Healthy SPECT Scan

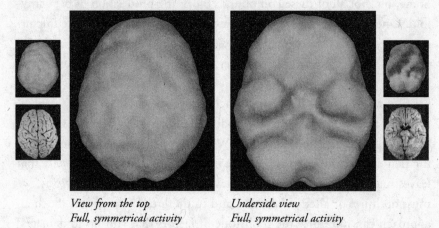

View from the top
Full, symmetrical activity

Underside view
Full, symmetrical activity

Note: *The small icons shown in the figures will be used throughout the text to help readers understand the orientation of the scans and how they differ from normal.*

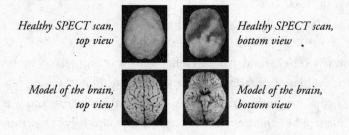

Healthy SPECT scan,
top view

Healthy SPECT scan,
bottom view

Model of the brain,
top view

Model of the brain,
bottom view

standardized set of blood tests to diagnose treatable conditions that mimic AD. She also underwent a brain SPECT scan, a sophisticated study that evaluates brain activity. The computerized screening battery and SPECT scan showed early signs of a serious problem. The SPECT scan showed decreased activity in the temporal lobes and parietal lobes (a hallmark finding for AD, as we will discuss in subsequent chapters).

Figures 1.3-4. Stacey's SPECT Scan

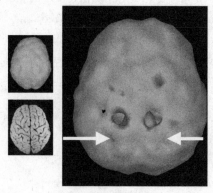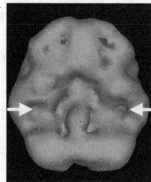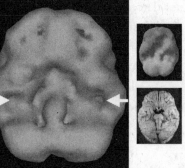

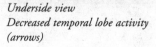

View from the top
Mild, decreased parietal lobe
activity (arrows)

Underside view
Decreased temporal lobe activity
(arrows)

Stacey followed the prevention and treatment strategies for AD explained in this book, which consisted of drug therapy with a cholinesterase inhibitor, low-dose vitamins E (200 IU a day) and C, daily physical exercise, and increased structure in her daily schedule. Within two months, she dramatically improved in her ability to teach her classes and remember recent events, and no longer had problems driving to new and old locations. Her confidence greatly improved, she became more aware of the difficulties that she had been previously experiencing, and her husband's stress and concern were greatly relieved. Jacqueline and her siblings were counseled on their risk factors for AD and given clear instructions on the best ways to fend off and delay AD.

An early diagnosis of AD presents bad news and good news. The bad news is that no one wants a diagnosis of a terrible disease with no known cure that erodes the brain, mind, and personality. The good news is that if it is caught in the earliest stages, prevention and treatment interventions have their best chance of working to delay the ravages of the disease.

Stacey's case is not an uncommon example of what can happen with prevention and early diagnosis and treatment of AD using the principles outlined in this book. Unfortunately, 95 percent of mildly demented people, such as Stacey, and 75 percent of moderately demented people are not detected by primary care physicians. Furthermore, standardized diagnostic criteria are not used by 75 percent of primary care physicians, so one can not simply rely on the family doctor to deal with this devastating problem. Awareness and embracing of *prevention through delay* is key.

While a diagnosis of Alzheimer's can be devastating, the earlier it is detected the more likely it is that, if it is treated properly, you and your family can avoid suffering the full-blown effects of the disease.

chapter   2

The Healthy Brain

The brain is the most complex and powerful organ in the universe. It is the command-and-control center of your life. It makes you who you are. It senses and integrates your inner world and the world around you. It produces your thoughts, feelings, memories, forethoughts, and actions. It is the organ of learning, loving, and working. Although it represents only about 2 percent of your body's weight (about 3 pounds), it uses 20 percent of the calories you consume. The brain uses its over 100 billion neurons to perceive and analyze incoming information; decides what, if anything, to do about the information; and then instructs the body to do it. To understand a troubled brain that leads to memory loss, we must first look at the healthy brain.

Neurons in Action

The brain, like other organs in the body, is made up of a collection of cells. In the brain the primary working cell is called a neuron or nerve cell. A neuron, like other cells, is enclosed in a membrane, has a nucleus that contains the genetic material, and is powered by energy packs called mitochondria. Unlike other cells, a neuron has two kinds of extensions from its membrane. One type are dendrites, which look like bushes or trees; a neuron typically has several main branches of dendrites. The other type is an *axon,* usually one to a neuron, which branches 10,000 to 40,000 times. Incoming information enters the neuron through dendrites, and outgoing information leaves the neuron through the axon. Dendrites and axons can grow and be modified throughout life, depending on experience.

A neuron's main job is to generate an electrical signal, called an action potential; it does this if it is sufficiently excited by other neurons. The action potential of a single neuron is like a lightning bolt that may stimulate many other neurons. The stimulated neurons can then generate their own action potentials that travel to and stimulate yet other neurons to which they are connected, creating a network of neurons that perform a specific brain function. Action potentials travel down axons at about 60 miles per hour. The signals can travel at these high speeds because axons are wrapped and insulated in a special protein called myelin. Axons that are not insulated by myelin, either by design or disease, transmit signals 10 times slower.

An axon branches 10,000 to 40,000 times, with each branch forming an electrical or chemical contact, called a synapse, to another neuron. The synaptic space is the tiny area between connecting neurons. At the end of each of the axon's many branches is a mushroom-shaped terminal, which contains molecules called neurotransmitters. These can excite or quiet other neurons. Each neuron makes a single type of neurotransmitter, such as glutamate, gamma-aminobuytric acid (GABA), dopamine, norepinephrine, serotonin, acetylcholine, or histamine. The primary excitatory neurotransmitter, glutamate, is released by 75 percent of all neurons in the brain, and the primary inhibitory neurotransmitter, GABA, is released by about 20 percent of all neurons in the brain. When the action potential reaches the end of the axon, it stimulates the release of thousands of neurotransmitter molecules into the synaptic space. The neurotransmitters float across this space, and some of them will bind to receptors on the receiving end of neurons and may stimulate or inhibit action of the receiving neuron.

Certain Parts of the Brain Tend to Do Specific Things

The brain is divided into four main lobes or regions: frontal, temporal, parietal and occipital (see Fig. 2.1). A useful generalization about how the brain functions is that the back half—the parietal lobe, the occipital lobe, and the back part of the temporal lobes—takes in and perceives the world. The front half of the brain integrates this information, analyzes it, decides what to do, and then plans and executes the decision. All four lobes can be involved in dementia. A brief summary of their functions and problems follows.

Frontal and Prefrontal Cortex

The frontal lobes (the front half of the brain) contain three important areas: the motor cortex, which controls the body's motor movements (such as walking, chewing, and moving your fingers and toes); the premotor

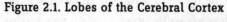

Figure 2.1. Lobes of the Cerebral Cortex

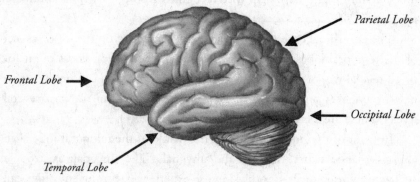

Frontal Lobe

Parietal Lobe

Occipital Lobe

Temporal Lobe

Left side view of brain

area, which is involved in planning motor movements, and the prefrontal cortex (PFC), which is intimately involved with executive functions such as planning, organizing, making judgments, exercising impulse control, and expressing what is on one's mind.

The PFC is the most evolved part of the human brain, representing 30 percent of its total mass, compared to that of the chimpanzee, our closest primate cousin, which occupies only 11 percent, or that of a dog's, only 7 percent, or that of a cat's, only 3.5 percent. The prefrontal cortex is responsible for the success and primacy of the human species. It houses our ability to learn from mistakes, make plans, and consistently match our behavior over time to reach our goals. When the PFC works as it should, we are thoughtful, empathic, able to express feelings appropriately, organized, and goal-directed.

Problems with the PFC result in poor judgment, impulsivity, short attention span, disorganization, trouble learning from experience, confusion, poor time management, and lack of empathy. These problems are often seen first in a type of ADRD called frontal-temporal lobe dementia and late in Alzheimer's disease.

Temporal Lobes

The temporal lobes, underneath your temples and behind your eyes, are involved with receptive language (hearing and reading), reading social cues, short-term memory, getting memories into long-term storage, and mood stability. They also help with recognizing objects by sight and naming them.

The entorhinal cortex and hippocampus, situated on the inside aspect of the temporal lobes, encode newly learned information and store it for up to several weeks. When these areas are damaged, you can neither store new experiences nor retrieve experiences learned within the past several weeks. These areas are the first to be damaged by AD.

In front of the hippocampus on the inside of the temporal lobe is an almond-shaped structure called the amygdala. The amygdala is strongly activated by fear, anger, or other intense experiences. Strong emotions can improve the encoding process of hippocampal neurons and make it easier to retrieve the experience. This is useful because it allows you to more easily remember events that were "emotionally stimulating," such as being mugged, having good sex, or recalling a fascinating fact you recently heard. By emphasizing the storage and memory of certain experiences over others, the amygdala allow you to respond more appropriately and quickly in the future; being able to recognize a potential mugger could save your life. When the amygdala fires the way it should, we tend to react to the world in a logical and thoughtful way. When it is overactive, we may overreact to the external events. When it is underactive, we fail to read situations accurately, and our response may not match what has happened. For example, if you laugh upon hearing from your wife that her best friend died, your amygdala may not be working properly. The undersides of the temporal lobes enable you to recognize people's faces.

Temporal lobe damage leads to short- and long-term memory problems, reading difficulties, trouble finding the right words in conversation, categorizing and comprehension difficulties, trouble reading social cues, episodes of rage, and religious or moral preoccupation.

Parietal Lobes

The parietal lobes are called the sensory brain, as they perceive light touch, pressure, vibration, pain, and temperature. They allow you to recognize objects by their feel, such as a comb or penny placed in your hand. The right parietal lobe perceives information from the left side of the body, while the left parietal lobe senses the right side. Farther back in the parietal lobes, important aspects of visual processing are performed, such as seeing motion and tracking objects in space (such as a kite or a football). They are involved with direction sense, the ability to know where you are in space, knowing right from left, and reading and creating maps in your mind. In addition, the parietal lobes help you understand what you read, perform basic symbolic operations involved in math (adding, subtracting, etc.), and allow you to mentally rotate objects in your mind.

The parietal lobes are damaged in AD after it spreads from the temporal lobes. Because the parietal lobes are heavily involved with direction sense, people with AD have trouble with directions, driving, getting lost, or losing their way. They may lose position sense and visual tracking, which means they may drop glasses, have trouble parking the car, or become confused when trying to put objects together (such as a model car). They also may experience trouble dressing, left-right confusion, trouble with math or writing, and impaired copying, drawing, or cutting. Denial or neglect of problems is another symptom of impaired parietal lobes, which prevents people from recognizing that they might have a serious problem, such as with driving or communicating.

Occipital Lobes

The occipital lobes, located at the back of the brain, process visual information. They process color, size, lines, and depth. In mapping vision, light first enters the retina of the eye, stimulating the optic nerve. The left half of your visual world crosses over to the right side of the brain to the primary visual cortex in the occipital lobes. Here light and shade are sorted out, color is perceived, and basic elements of vision (such as lines, shapes, and angles) are perceived.

From the occipital lobes, the part of the visual information involved in recognizing what you see moves to the temporal lobes. The part of visual processing that follows the motion of objects goes from the occipital to the parietal lobes.

Damage to the occipital lobes may cause changes in sight and perception and lead to visual hallucinations, illusions, or blindness. When one side of the occipital lobe is damaged, you can't see the opposite side of your environment. So if the left occipital lobe is damaged, you can't see things to your right. Damage in the occipital lobes can cause particularly interesting side effects. One of the strangest is blindsight. A person with blindsight claims that they have no vision at all but can recognize moving objects in the part of their visual field that is apparently blind. A type of dementia called Lewy body dementia (LBD) often starts with symptoms of occipital lobe damage in which hallucinations of dwarves or midgets are common.

Table 2.1. Brain Function Summary

	Prefrontal Cortex	Temporal Lobes	Parietal Lobes	Occipital Lobes
Functions				
	Judgment	Hearing/listening	Direction sense	Sight
	Impulse control	Reading	Sensory perception	Color perception
	Attention span	Reading social cues, include speech tone	Spatial processing, sees motion	Lines
	Organization	Short-term memory	Visual guidance, such as to grab objects	Depth
	Self-monitoring	Long-term memory	Recognize objects by touch	
	Problem solving	Recognizing objects by sight	Ability to know where you are in space	
	Critical thinking	Anger control	Know right from left	
	Empathy	Naming things	Reading and creating maps	
Problems				
	Poor judgment	Short-term memory loss	Impaired direction sense	Visual problems
	Impulsivity	Reading problems	Trouble dressing or putting objects together	Can't see outlines of objects
	Short attention	Word-finding problems	Left-right confusion	Visual (simple) hallucination
	Disorganization	Trouble reading social cues	Denial of illness	Visual illusions (simple)
	Trouble learning from experience	Episodic rage	Impaired position sense	Blindsight
	Confusion	Poor object recognition	Trouble with math or writing	Functional blindness
	Poor time management		Neglect or unawareness of what you see	Objects appear larger or smaller than they are
	Repeated mistakes	Religious or moral preoccupation	Impaired copying, drawing, or cutting	Colors not recognized
	Lack of empathy			

What the Brain Needs to Stay Healthy

Fuel

Just like any other living thing, a brain needs fuel to grow, function, and repair itself. Glucose and oxygen run the engine powered by your brain cells. Glucose is a simple six-carbon sugar. Unlike other cells in your body, your brain cells only know how to use glucose. Anything that impairs glucose delivery to brain cells is life-threatening. Oxygen is required to produce energy; without it your mitochondria will not produce enough energy to keep your brain alive. Because blood delivers glucose and oxygen to your brain, nothing must get in the way of blood flow if the brain is to stay healthy.

Stimulation

Although largely genetically programmed to turn on its functions at the right developmental age, the human brain also depends on proper stimulation to grow and develop throughout childhood and to maintain its functioning into old age. When you stimulate neurons in the right way, you make them more efficient; they function better, and you are more likely to have an active, learning brain throughout your life. The physiology of stimulation is called long-term potentiation (LTP). This refers to the process of invigorating (or potentiating) neurons to do their job efficiently. It is accomplished, quite simply, through the repetition of an act, which causes actual physical changes in neurons and their synapses.

Long-term potentiation causes the nerve endings to get bigger, which creates a significant advantage on two fronts. First, they are harder to damage. Second, the larger surface area on the neurons allows for more electrochemical signals to pass between cells, enhancing efficient communication. In the process of potentiation, receiving neurons can generate their own signals with less input in the future; this means that once LTP has occurred it takes less energy to do something well. For instance, a pianist who has been practicing a piece by Mozart will be able, after a year, to play it without struggle, without thinking about it, because she has been steadily stimulating the synapses on the neurons that control her finger movements so they can execute the proper sequence to play the piece. She has "potentiated" her neurons in just the right way to accomplish that goal.

The *way* the pianist practices makes all the difference, because the brain does not interpret what it receives; it simply translates it. The brain doesn't care if the person is becoming a great piano player or a terrible piano player. Consequently, if she is repeating imperfect fingering, she will become very good at playing imperfectly. If she is training herself to be a perfect pianist, it is essential that she practices perfectly, that she not learn bad habits or sloppy fingering of the keys, and that she work with a professional who can correct her mistakes. Her brain doesn't care what she gives it, so if *she* cares whether she plays well or badly, she must be certain that she is giving her brain the right training.

The best sources of stimulation for the brain are physical exercise, mental exercise, and social bonding.

Physical Exercise

Physical exercise is important for brain health. Moderate exercise improves the heart's ability to pump blood throughout the body and helps maintain healthy blood flow to the brain, which increases oxygen and glucose delivery. Exercise also reduces damage to neurons from toxic substances from the environment, and it enhances insulin's ability to prevent high blood sugar levels, thereby reducing the risk of diabetes. Physical exercise also helps protect the short-term memory structures in the temporal lobes (hippocampus and entorhinal cortex) from high-stress conditions, which produce excessive amounts of the hormone cortisol (20). In fact, some persons with Alzheimer's disease have higher cortisol levels than normal aging persons (21). Physical exercise makes the whole body healthier. It does this by improving the tone of the blood vessels, which decreases the risk for high blood pressure, stroke, and heart disease and increases blood flow to all the organs in the body to make them hardier. In addition, it helps maintain coordination, agility, and speed. The Honolulu Study of Aging found that untreated high blood pressure during midlife (40 to 60 years old) greatly increases the risk for dementia. For middle-aged persons with a systolic blood pressure of 160 mm Hg or higher, or a diastolic blood pressure of 90 mm Hg or higher, the risk of dementia after age 70 was 3.8 to 4.8 times greater than those whose high blood pressure was treated (22). This study emphasizes the importance of regular exercise and proper treatment of any medical conditions you may have.

Exercise actually stimulates "neurogenesis," the ability of the brain to generate new neurons. In exercising laboratory rats, research shows that they generate new neurons in the frontal lobe and hippocampus that survive for about four weeks and then die off unless they are stimulated (23). If you stimulate these new neurons through mental or social interaction, then they connect to other neurons and become integrated into brain circuits that help maintain their functions throughout your life. Exercise provides the raw materials. The brain needs to grow and repair itself. Reading, playing music, creating art, writing, and other "mental" pastimes strengthen and grow the specific brain areas used.

Lack of exercise negatively affects blood supply in the body. A molecule in the cell walls of blood vessels called nitric oxide controls the shape of blood vessels throughout the body. If it does not receive pulses of blood flow on a regular basis from exercise, the blood vessel walls begin to distort and block the flow of blood through the vessel, which means that the person is not maintaining good oxygenation and glucose delivery. If the deep areas of the brain are starved of these nutrients, the person will have problems coordinating his limbs and with processing complex thoughts. A regular habit of physical exercise is a major preventive strategy for Alzheimer's disease and related disorders (18). The Sydney Older Persons Study found that exercise levels in persons 75 years and older did not reduce risk of Alzheimer's disease or other causes of dementia (24). This means that it is important to establish a regular habit of exercise in your life now, and not wait until your seventies to start.

Mental Exercise

Physical exercise has a global effect on the brain, but mental exercise is equally important. By mental exercise, we mean acquiring new knowledge. It is possible to use your brain without learning anything new, which in the long run is not terribly helpful. For instance, Dr. Joe L. reads mammograms all day long—reads thousands of them a year—and although he is working his brain every day, he is not actually taking in new information. Whenever the brain does something over and over, it learns how to do that particular thing using less and less energy. New learning—such as learning a new medical technique, a new hobby, or new game—helps establish new connections, thus maintaining and improving the function of other less-often-used brain areas.

The famous Religious Orders study is an important example of the power of this "Use it or lose it" principle of mental exercise. In this study, Robert Wilson, Ph.D., and colleagues examined the frequency of mentally stimulating activities, such as reading a newspaper, among 801 older nuns, priests, and other clergy over five years. The study discovered that those who increased their mental activity over the five years reduced their chance of developing Alzheimer's disease by one-third. These more mentally active people also reduced their age-related decline in overall mental abilities by 50 percent, in concentration and attention span by 60 percent, and in mental processing speed by 30 percent (25).

Taking classes to learn about new and interesting subjects or finding a job that requires you to learn new skills will stimulate brain growth. Both of these activities activate the short-term memory areas of the brain (the hippocampus and the entorhinal cortex) and require one to use the judgment (in the frontal lobe) to select what to learn.

Some repetitive mental stimulation can be helpful; common activities such as gardening, sewing, playing bridge, reading, painting, and doing crossword puzzles have value. These activities protect the specific abilities involved in performing that particular mental exercise from declining if the person does get AD. A good example is Alan Jay Lerner of the Lerner and Loew musical team. After years of writing brilliant lyrics, for musicals such as *Brigadoon, My Fair Lady, Camelot,* and *Paint Your Wagon,* Lerner developed Alzheimer's disease and became severely demented. He could not tell people his name or his address, but well into his nineties he could play every piece of music he ever wrote. The circuits he most frequently used during his lifetime for playing the piano and writing musical scores were well protected against dementia.

Even with an activity that one is used to doing all the time, it is still possible to learn something new. Learning a new technique or approach will stimulate your hippocampus and entorhinal cortex to become more resistant to different kinds of brain damage. A major exception to this rule is the "activity" of watching TV, which may actually increase the risk of AD in persons who watch two or more hours a day, as shown by a recent study. However, this study did not specify whether watching programs that teach you something had the same effect as pure entertainment, such as situation comedies. We suspect that passively watching TV is the problem and that watching TV to actively learn something may not only not increase the chance of AD but even reduce the risk.

Learning has a very real effect on neurons: it keeps them firing and it makes it easier for them to fire. There are approximately a thousand trillion synapses in the brain, and each one of them may wither away if not actively firing. Like muscles that don't get used, they atrophy. The brain has many, many different circuits. Any set of circuits that does not get used grows weak. For example, middle-aged people who go back to college often feel mentally slow at first, and it takes a few semesters of mental exercise before they find academic studies easy again. What is also at work here is that with age, the level of activity of the enzymes in one's cells starts to decline. The cells become less efficient, and one's brain isn't quite as agile as that of an 18-year-old. However, in some ways, younger people are at a disadvantage. In certain respects, the 50-year-old will do better in academic studies because as one ages, one's frontal lobes are better developed. As the executive part of the brain, the frontal lobes are involved in judgment, forethought, and impulse control, which usually helps a person pay better attention in class and ask better questions. A more developed frontal lobe allows you to take better advantage of new knowledge, to know what to focus on, and to relate it to your life experiences so that it has more useful value to you. The 18-year-old may be able to memorize facts easier, but her frontal lobe isn't as good at selecting *which* facts to memorize.

Social Interaction

One common source of brain stimulation that is often overlooked is interacting with other people. Social interaction is the fuel the brain needs to develop the ability to negotiate, cooperate, and compromise with others, to know right from wrong, and to know when to respond and when to keep silent. These highly complex human abilities are largely controlled by the tips of the frontal lobes. They start to develop before two years old, such as when the infant starts saying no to the parents. These abilities continue to develop at least until 50 years old, according to studies of brain myelination, and perhaps longer.

Child neglect has been associated with many brain-based developmental difficulties such as personality and learning and behavioral problems. Likewise, adults deprived of the company of others experience a clear negative effect on cognitive abilities, memory, and social skills. In studies on social connectedness in the elderly, it has been shown that people who spend time with others on a regular basis are cognitively sharper. In addition, their emotions are more even. Psychiatrists have seen time and again that people who are isolated commit suicide dramatically more often than those who are active in society. Simple social interaction stimulates particular neuronal circuits. For instance, there is a self-awareness circuit at the very tip of the frontal lobe. If its capacity is diminished, the person can no longer judge her own abilities. Self-awareness is maintained, literally, by being aware of oneself, and that is aided significantly by feedback from other people. If the circuits in the crucial areas of the frontal lobe aren't being used, they atrophy, and the person's social skills suffer.

The Birth, and Death, of Brain Cells

The brain not only has to grow, develop, and mature but also has to repair itself on a constant basis. It's not like a car that you can take into a garage when it needs a tune-up or when it has to have a part replaced. Your brain has mechanisms to repair damage as a result of the normal wear and tear of life. The hardware of the brain—neurons, their dendrites, axons, and synapses, as well as glial cells, which help support and nourish neurons—has to be maintained.

The brain has to maintain its 100 billion neurons to consistently function well. If the number of neurons in any cortical circuit decreases by more than one-third, the circuit can no longer compensate for the loss, and dysfunction of that circuit appears. In Alzheimer's disease, the earliest damage occurs in the hippocampus and entorhinal cortex of the temporal lobe and does not spread to other areas for somewhere between 10 and 50 years (26). When the first symptoms of AD finally appear, they are only related to these damaged areas—namely, occasional lapses of short-term memory—that are often attributed to "just getting older." The individual's symptoms therefore tell a specialist which areas of the brain have been damaged.

It is still commonly believed that we are born with all of the nerve cells we will ever have and that human brains simply cannot replace dead neurons. Because of this, scientists used to consider brain damage irreversible and neurological disease in the elderly unstoppable. In stunning new research, investigators have discovered that adult human brains generate the DNA needed to make new nerve cells in the brain. Since then, scientists have been furiously studying the implications, and research in this area has accelerated.

Neurogenesis means birth, but the birth cycle is begun by death. Let's say you go to a New Year's Eve party and have a little too much champagne. You come home and sleep it off. By the time you awake, several hundred thousand neurons have died from alcohol toxicity. Somehow, the number of neurons in your brain has to be brought back up to normal to reach a *steady state*. Neurogenesis is the process that develops and maintains the functional capacity of the circuits by replacing neurons that are killed or damaged. The very act of the neurons dying triggers certain growth factors in the brain to stimulate the formation of new neurons. But neurogenesis doesn't know when to stop; left on its own, it will continue creating new neurons until the brain explodes. The brain has to regulate itself so that just the right numbers of neurons are maintained. When the number generated reaches a certain level, cell death is triggered, which miraculously brings the number back down. Yet once again, this death mechanism does not know when to stop killing, and thus new neuron formation is triggered again. This process allows brain cell growth to stay within a certain range, so that the circuits can always function well—at least under normal conditions.

This brain repair process is called synaptic plasticity, neurogenesis, and cell death. You can think of it simply as the brain's governor, whose main job is to govern the population. It must maintain the right balance or all hell will break loose. Not only do the numbers of cells have to be regulated but so do the one thousand trillion synapses that connect them. It is essential for brain function to maintain synaptic health.

How Diseases Impair Brain Function

With this basic understanding of how the brain works, one can now see that a *disease will impair a specific brain function by preventing action potentials from successfully traveling through the network of synaptically connected neurons that generate that function.* Diseases can:

- Reduce the number of neurons in a network, which happens in Alzheimer's disease (initially in the temporal and parietal lobes) and seizure disorders (often in the temporal lobes)
- Reduce the number of synapses in a network, which happens when there is depression or a lack of mental or physical exercise
- Impair the generation of action potentials, which can happen if one consumes three or more alcoholic drinks at a time
- Disrupt cell body machinery to block action potential generation, which happens in Parkinson's disease, diabetes, and chemotherapy and radiation therapy for cancer
- Damage axons to slow the speed of action potentials and reduce the chance that they will successfully travel through the whole network, as in hypertension, heart disease, strokes, and head trauma

chapter 3

Seven Ways to Lose Your Mind: How Memory Loss Starts

The phrase *Alzheimer's disease and related disorders* (ADRD) is used to define a group of diseases that have one thing in common: each is a cause of mild cognitive impairment (MCI) or dementia. *Dementia* is defined as a progressive condition with two or more impairments in mental skills that interfere with a person's ability to function in his usual manner in his social, family, personal, or professional life. Just as delayed diagnosis and treatment of high blood pressure, diabetes, heart disease, stroke, and most other diseases leads to less effective treatment results, the same holds for delayed diagnosis and treatment of ADRD.

Dementing diseases start by affecting a very small amount of brain, usually in just one location. Each dementing disease tends to start in its own distinctive location, and it can take years before enough brain damage has amassed to produce the first symptom. The specific symptom produced depends on which brain area is damaged. As long as only one symptom exists, the condition is classified as MCI; this is the stage at which ADRD diseases are most clearly distinct from one another. If the disease causing MCI is not diagnosed and treated effectively, it will progress and affect other brain areas. Once enough damage accumulates in these other brain areas, additional symptoms will appear, and the dementia syndrome has begun. With further progression of the dementia, ADRD diseases share more and more of the same symptoms. The affected brains also start to look the same when they are imaged. By the time dementia has become moderate or severe, diagnosing its cause is much more difficult.

Detecting ADRD Early

The most effective prevention and treatment strategies require a correct diagnosis, which is easier to make in the early stages of ADRD. We all know that detecting cancer early can lead to a longer, healthier, and more pain-free life. The same is true of detecting diabetes early, when the only finding is an elevated blood sugar level. Diabetics detected early and treated effectively can live a full, healthy life *even though their diabetes isn't actually "cured."* The majority of ADRD diseases are no different. Early detection and treatment of ADRD, including Alzheimer's disease, may delay symptoms long enough to allow you to live out your life independently, not become a burden on your family, and not have to be put into a nursing home. For ADRD, delaying the onset and progression of dementia symptoms so long that you live most of your natural life unaffected by them translates practically into a cure.

Despite tremendous advances in ADRD treatment, 95 percent of persons with ADRD are diagnosed four years after the first symptoms appear (27). By that time they are moderately demented and completely dependent on others for their care. Detecting ADRD this late is equivalent to diagnosing a diabetic when she is blind, has kidney failure, and can no longer feel her limbs. Thanks to annual screening for diabetes, hypertension, heart disease, cancer, and many other chronic diseases of aging, in most persons these diseases are detected early and treated effectively. Given

Table 3.1. The Most Common Causes of Mild Cognitive Impairment and ADRD

1. Degenerative Brain Diseases

Alzheimer's disease
Lewy body disease
Parkinson's disease
Frontal-temporal lobe diseases

2. Vascular Brain Diseases

Large strokes
Multiple strokes
Strokes in deep brain areas

3. Cancer and Cancer Treatments

Primary brain tumors
Metastases from other cancers to the brain
Chemotherapy
Radiation therapy

4. Head Trauma

5. Infectious and Immunological Diseases

Multiple sclerosis (MS)
Chronic fatigue immunodeficiency syndrome (CFIDS)
Creutzfeld-Jakob Disease (CJD, or "mad cow disease")
Herpes viruses
Human immunodeficiency viruses (HIV, the virus that causes AIDS)
Brain infections (meningitis, encephalitis, abscess)

6. Alcohol and Other Brain Toxins

7. Disorders Affecting Nerve Cell Metabolism

Depression
Thyroid diseases
Diabetes
Hypoglycemia
Kidney diseases
Liver diseases
Lung diseases
Hydrocephalus (normal pressure, obstructive and nonobstructive types)
Seizures (epilepsy)
Hypoxia
B vitamin deficiencies (B_{12}, thiamine, or folic acid)
High calcium levels
High homocysteine levels
Estrogen deficiency
Testosterone deficiency
High or low cortisol levels

that we can detect ADRD early and that early treatment can greatly improve the rest of one's life, why should detecting ADRD late be acceptable to anyone, given its devastating consequences?

Although ADRD treatment is usually effective, it is not *perceived* to be so because most patients start treatment when they have end-stage disease. Starting treatment in the end stage of any disease is usually ineffective; this is not peculiar to ADRD. In the case of ADRD, however, *delayed detection of dementia leads to delayed treatment and being put in a nursing home.* The fear of this outcome causes people to avoid getting screened for ADRD until it is too late.

The first step in applying the concept of *prevention through delay* is to understand how memory loss starts and the seven ways you can lose your mind (see Table 3.1).

Because of space constraints, we cannot cover every one of these illnesses, but will examine the most common ones.

Degenerative Brain Diseases

Degenerative diseases directly damage certain brain areas by destroying neurons or their supporting cells. Up to a point, the brain's repair processes can keep up with this damage. Eventually, degenerative diseases will cause more damage than can be repaired, and the numbers of neurons begin to decline. However, the symptoms related to a damaged brain area do not appear until its number of neurons declines by about one-third (28). For example, it takes between 10 and 50 years of damage to the entorhinal cortex—the first brain area affected by Alzheimer's disease—before the first symptom, memory loss for recent events, appears. At this time, between 30 and 60 percent of the neurons in the entorhinal cortex have been lost (29).

When a symptom first appears, it may only be occasional, as when you are under a lot of pressure or stress. You may go somewhere and not remember having been there before, even though it was *memorable*. You may not remember a conversation a few days ago that was important to you. Over time, as the disease continues to destroy brain cells, the symptom will consistently appear.

All types of degenerative diseases usually begin after age 40, because cells are then more susceptible to damage and death. After age 40, your body produces less energy because of a slower metabolism. Consequently, cells are less able to produce antioxidants, which soak up free radicals (a waste product of cell activity) and prevent them from killing cells.

Programmed cell death, or apoptosis, is one important mechanism by which free radicals kill cells. Free radicals can turn on specific proteins in cells that activate death genes, which instruct cells to literally commit suicide. Apoptosis is known to occur in Alzheimer's disease, Parkinson's disease, Lewy body disease, frontal temporal lobe disease, Huntington's disease, stroke, epilepsy, and many other disorders.

Degenerative brain diseases are often due to a combination of genetic and behavioral factors. There is usually a tendency to develop a disease due to particular genes you inherit: *diseases run in families*. There are also behavioral or lifestyle patterns that predispose you to develop that disease. Changing these patterns can not only lower your risk from the lifestyle factor, it can also lower genetic risk. The most dramatic example of this gene-behavior interaction is with Alzheimer's disease in Africans. The E4 version (allele) of the apolipoprotein E gene is the major genetic risk factor for inheriting the late-onset type of Alzheimer's disease, which usually produces symptoms after the age of 60 (see Chapter 5). Africans living in America who have the apolipoprotein E4 allele have the expected increased risk of Alzheimer's disease. However, Africans living below the Sahara who have the apolipoprotein E4 allele actually have a reduced risk of developing Alzheimer's disease. One major difference between these two groups of Africans is that those living in sub-Saharan Africa get lots of exercise and eat low-fat diets. The apolipoprotein E4 allele also increases risk for heart disease and stroke due to hardening of the arteries by increasing levels of low-density lipoprotein (the LDL in the fasting cholesterol blood test). Exercise and diet in these "at-risk Africans" actually reduce the effects of the E4 allele to lower that risk for developing Alzheimer's disease.

The most common of the degenerative brain diseases that cause MCI and dementia are the following four: Alzheimer's disease, Lewy body disease, Parkinson's disease, and the frontal-temporal lobe diseases.

Alzheimer's Disease

Alzheimer's disease (AD) was first described in 1906 by the German physician Alois Alzheimer after evaluating, treating, and eventually autopsying a 50-year-old woman. Her husband had complained that his wife had serious memory problems and that she relentlessly (and inaccurately) accused him of being unfaithful. Dr. Alzheimer found that the patient could recognize and describe common objects, but their names eluded her. When she was shown a cup, for instance, she described it as a milk jug. And then, several minutes later, she did not remember seeing the cup at all. Because of the naming problem, she frequently stopped midsentence, unable to find the right words to express herself. Upon her death, Dr. Alzheimer examined her brain using a newly developed high-resolution microscope. He found "peculiar formations" outside of neurons and "dense tangled bundles" within them. These lesions are now known to be the signature neuritic plaques (outside neurons) and neurofibrillary tangles (within neurons) of Alzheimer's disease (30).

It is commonly thought that AD evolves in five stages, as follows.

Stage 1 lasts 10 to 50 years; AD lesions are only found in the entorhinal cortex, on the inside of the temporal lobes. No symptoms of short-term memory loss occur because less than one-third of the entorhinal cortex has been damaged.

Stage 2 lasts two to four years. More than one-third of the entorhinal cortex is damaged, and AD has spread into the adjacent area called the hippocampus. Damage is severe enough to block the encoding and storing of new experiences, events, or conversations so that they cannot be recalled minutes to weeks later (short-term memory loss). This stage is when mild cognitive impairment (MCI) begins. During Stage 2, the damage also spreads from the entorhinal cortex to connected areas of the brain that integrate your emotions and experiences. Consequently, mood-related symptoms of apathy, anger, fear, anxiety, and social withdrawal can appear in Stage 2.

Stage 3 lasts two to eight years. Mild dementia begins when AD lesions spread to still other areas, called the association cortex, in the parietal and temporal lobes. The association cortex literally associates different types of information from cortical areas that do simpler things such as identify the curvature of someone's face, the color of her eyes, or the sound of her voice. The association cortex performs complex functions such as recognizing a friend, recalling her name, and tracking her movement. When AD damages more than one-third of an association cortical area, its function becomes impaired. Related symptoms then appear, such as having greater difficulty retrieving the right words to describe something, recognizing the face of someone you know, or understanding conversations.

Stage 4 lasts two to six years. Moderate dementia begins when AD lesions in the association cortex spread to connected brain areas in the frontal lobes. The frontal lobes take the auditory, visual, and tactile information from the parietal and temporal association cortex, plus the information from the emotional brain, and integrate them together to create the whole experience for you. When we meet someone and talk with him, we don't only perceive the color of his eyes; we perceive everything about him all at once, including his eye color, the shape of his face and body, the sound of his voice, the meaning of his words, the emotion expressed behind them, and so on, which is one of the functions of your frontal lobes. When AD damages more than one-third of a frontal lobe area, then the kinds of symptoms that develop relate to *misinterpreting the whole experience*. Examples of such misinterpretation include (1) seeing shadows outside your window and interpreting them to be burglars; (2) feeling tingling over your stomach and interpreting it to be bugs crawling on you; and (3) a wife seeing her husband with a female friend and interpreting them to be having an affair. When the person cannot be convinced that his or her interpretations are wrong, they have what are called paranoid delusions. Persons can express paranoia as fearfulness, anxiety, terror, anger, suspicion, social withdrawal, or depression.

Stage 5 lasts two to four years. Severe dementia begins when the disease becomes widespread, for example to the area of the brain called the primary motor cortex. Everything you *do* is executed by the primary motor cortex. Things as simple as drinking, eating, brushing teeth, bathing, dressing, toileting, and walking are all executed by the primary motor cortex. When things go wrong in this part of the brain, people have trouble with (1) falling and fracturing a hip; (2) choking and developing pneumonia; and (3) losing control of urine and developing a bladder infection. These symptoms usually lead to infection and death in AD.

What Causes Alzheimer's Disease?

It is thought that there are two primary processes that cause AD: the accumulation of toxic beta amyloid plaques and the formation of neurofibrillary tangles inside neurons.

Beta Amyloid Plaques   Amyloid precursor protein (APP) is a normal protein (a protein is a string of amino acids) necessary for brain development and repair. After it is used, APP gets broken down into a harmless 37-amino-acid fragment, which is then recycled into more APP. People with Alzheimer's disease, though, have significantly higher levels of one of two enzymes, the beta and gamma secretases, which break down APP into a 40- or 42-amino-acid fragment, both of which are called beta amyloid. This 42-amino-acid fragment (BA42) is believed to be a major cause of the disease process in AD.

The BA42 fragments combine with salt and water in the brain to cre-

Figure 3.1 Normal v. Abnormal Plaques in the Brain

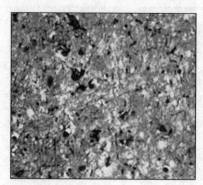

No neuritic plaques

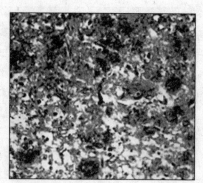

Image loaded with neuritic plaques

ate a sticky mess of crisscrossing proteins (BA42 complexes). These complexes damage the brain in two ways. First, normal plaques, which consist of harmless breakdown products that accumulate with age (like aging spots on your skin), are invaded by BA42 complexes, which convert them into deadly neuritic plaques. Neuritic plaques disrupt the brain's normal repair process, causing short circuits to accumulate and resulting in brain dysfunction. Second, BA42 complexes cause too much calcium to enter neurons, which overexcites them and turns on death genes that program neurons to commit suicide (apoptosis).

Neurofibrillary Tangles   The second primary process occurs within the cells themselves. Proteins called *tau* normally form the neuron's basic shape and backbone. Microscopically, they look like steel girders that give the neuron its characteristic shape. Mutations of a gene on chromosome 17 have been found to cause the tau protein to twist, blocking the flow of molecules from the cell body to the outer regions, causing the cell to wither and die. With AD, there is a significant increase in these tangled filaments, or neurofibrillary tangles (NFTs), which accumulate inside the neuron and block healthy activity.

Figure 3.2. Neurofibrillary Tangle Progression

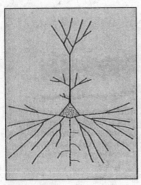 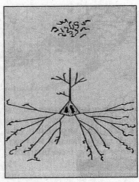 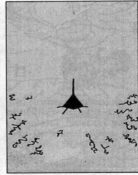

Normal neuron   *Early-stage NFT;*   *Late-stage NFT:*
                         note twisted dendrites   *a dead neuron*

Early Symptoms of AD

The first symptoms of Alzheimer's almost always arise because the person has trouble encoding new information or experiences. Most frequently, this manifests as forgetting appointments, names, taking your medication on time (particularly ones the doctor changed), significant family events or holidays, or locations you have recently visited.

Short-term memory loss can present itself in many other forms. One may find it hard to perform complex tasks, get lost when trying to visit a new place, or have trouble following directions about how to do something. Of all the eventual symptoms of Alzheimer's disease, short-term memory loss is usually the earliest, because the entorhinal cortex—the main bridge for getting memory into storage—is disrupted. It is now known that the earliest stage of neurofibrillary tangle development in AD begins in the entorhinal cortex.

The job of this brain area is to take in all aspects of whatever it is the person wants to remember and wrap them into one experience, a single package, before sending it along to the hippocampus for encoding. This flow of electrical-chemical activity, the purpose of which is to encode and store a recent event, represents a giant brain circuit. It starts in the brain areas that created the original perception of the event. Then it travels through the entorhinal cortex and hippocampus. Then it flows back to the entorhinal cortex. And finally, it returns to the original brain areas.

Damage to the entorhinal cortex creates a destructive traffic jam to the flow of this important circuit. A disruption of this order is something like being stuck in rush-hour traffic in the Holland Tunnel in New York City. This is why a problem with encoding a new experience is the first symptom; incoming information gets jammed in the tunnel (the entorhinal cortex) and cannot arrive at its true destination.

Spouses and friends of people with Alzheimer's disease often misinterpret their actions. They believe the person is intentionally selecting what to remember and what to forget. We have heard many spouses say, "My husband doesn't have a memory problem. He remembers everything we used to do throughout our marriage. He just doesn't want to remember what's happening now. And I know he's not listening to me because he asks the same question over and over. Either he's lost interest in our marriage or he is just in denial."

This kind of interpretation—that the forgetful person is doing it on purpose—causes considerable stress, hurt feelings, resentment, and anger in a marriage. Most of the time, it is just plain wrong. For a person to be in denial of information, she must know that something happened in the first place. However, in AD, the damage to the entorhinal cortex and hippocampus prevents new memories from being recorded. In other words, for all intents and purposes, the recent activity, conversation, or event never "occurred" because the brain did not record it or store it. Understanding this fundamental truth—that for persons with AD, recent events, experiences, and conversations simply never happened—can help families cope with their loved one's exasperating behavior.

The spouse's complaint that her husband remembered "everything we used to do" is accurate. With AD, in the early stages at least, long-term memories *are* preserved. The husband who can't remember what his wife said yesterday can still recall what she said on their honeymoon. An event that far in the past is stored in long-term memory, which is a network of neurons in other parts of the brain. To retrieve a memory of his honeymoon, the husband's brain does not need the entorhinal cortex and hippocampus (the short-term memory factories), so he can function in a reasonably normal way when retrieving events of long ago. Later on, as AD progresses into the other parts of the cerebral cortex, long-term memory becomes just as damaged as short-term memory, but in the early stages, the person can still retrieve memories from the distant past without too much trouble.

Diagnosing AD

Today's brain imaging methods can detect each stage of AD, helping tremendously with early detection, correct diagnosis, effective treatment, and proper monitoring.

Tony ❖ Detecting AD Before Symptoms Begin

Tony was a 59-year-old successful shopkeeper. He had no symptoms of his own and was not concerned about his own memory per se, but his mother had recently died of AD, and he wanted to find out about prevention in case he was at risk. He took Dr. Shankle's dementia screening tools (see Appendix A). Although neither Tony nor his wife perceived any problems with his memory, the testing revealed that his short-term memory was below normal for a person of his age, sex, and education. The test results recommended further evaluation.

Dr. Shankle ordered the recommended blood tests and imaging studies needed to accurately diagnose ADRD. The blood tests showed that Tony had one apolipoprotein E4 gene, which increased his risk for AD. The hospital's radiologist read Tony's brain MRI as normal but did not comment on the hippocampus and entorhinal cortex in the temporal lobe. Dr. Shankle reviewed the same MRI, which clearly showed a 25 percent loss of brain tissue in the entorhinal cortex and hippocampus. Unfortunately, many radiologists do not routinely inspect the hippocampus and entorhinal cortex when looking for early stage AD, even though it is the first place where tissue loss occurs in AD. A large number of early stage AD diagnoses are probably missed in this way. An MRI report cannot be relied on to exclude the diagnosis of AD if it has not specifically commented on whether there is tissue loss in the entorhinal cortex and hippocampus.

Figure 3.3. Tony's SPECT Study

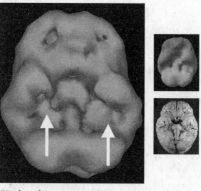

Underside view
Decreased activity in the temporal lobes

Dr. Shankle wanted to determine if any areas besides the hippocampus and entorhinal cortex had reduced brain activity, so he ordered a SPECT study. It showed reduced activity in the same areas as the MRI.

Because Tony's testing showed short-term memory loss, even though he and his wife were not aware of it, and because his MRI showed tissue loss in the entorhinal cortex and hippocampus only, he was diagnosed with Stage 2 AD. He is now being treated with the medication Exelon to help block neuritic plaque and neurofibrillary tangle formation, plus a combination of antioxidants to reduce the chance of programmed cell death (apoptosis). After six months, Tony's repeat testing showed that his short-term memory had improved.

In Tony's case, an MRI could have diagnosed AD if the radiologist had examined the hippocampus and entorhinal cortex for tissue loss. Tony was lucky for two reasons: first, he was already alerted to the fact that he might have a problem; and second, he had a SPECT scan that clearly showed the disease was still in its early stages (Stage 2 AD). The SPECT scan and office testing allowed us to measure the effects of the most up-to-date AD treatments to determine how well they were really working. Not only did his symptoms improve, the rate of progression of AD in his brain will be delayed for at least several years. By then, newer, more effective treatments will probably be available that will make it possible to stabilize Tony in his current state of having no symptoms for the rest of his life. Thus we can now offer a realistic chance that Tony and others like him will live their entire lives without suffering the symptoms of Alzheimer's disease, just as a diabetic or hypertensive person may never suffer the symptoms of diabetes or hypertension if the disease is detected early and treated effectively.

Tony's case truly represents *prevention through delay*, which would not have happened had his mother's death not alerted him to see a physician instead of waiting for symptoms to appear. This underscores the importance of an annual memory screen in all persons over age 50, starting earlier if family risk factors are present.

Lewy Body Disease (LBD)

This disease, initially described by the neurologist F. H. Lewy in 1912, accounts for 10–20 percent of MCI and dementia in older adults, usually over 70 years old. It is a degenerative disorder associated with abnormal deposits (Lewy bodies) found in certain areas of the brain. Lewy bodies contain deposits of a protein called alpha-synuclein, which is also linked to Parkinson's disease.

Early Symptoms

Early symptoms include those involving movement, visual perception, level of consciousness, and memory loss. Early LBD symptoms affecting movement are similar to Parkinson's disease symptoms. They include increasing difficulty with:

- Starting to move the body or limbs
- Moving as quickly as one had in the past
- Relaxing the muscles of the neck, arms, or legs
- Involuntary trembling of the head or limbs while at rest
- Walking, which is replaced by short, little steps like those of an infant
- Balance and posture, which leads to leaning and falling

Early LBD symptoms affecting visual perception are usually visual hallucinations due to Lewy bodies accumulating in the visual cortex in the occipital lobes of the brain. Dwarf-like people are often described and are quite vivid but not necessarily frightening.

Another early symptom that is often diagnostic of LBD is the response to medications that block the neurotransmitter dopamine. These medications, often referred to as antipsychotics or neuroleptics, are used to treat hallucinations in persons with schizophrenia but are also given to older individuals who have hallucinations. However, people with LBD have markedly reduced dopamine levels in their brains, which is the cause of their difficulty with movement. Giving a medication to an LBD person that further reduces dopamine can cause a marked worsening of his symptoms, making him rigid as a board and sometimes putting him into a coma.

Unfortunately, people with LBD sometimes do not recover from being given antipsychotic medication.

Early LBD symptoms affecting level of consciousness include confusion and drowsiness during the daytime, or sleep disturbances at night, and are due to Lewy bodies accumulating in brainstem pathways that maintain consciousness. Studies have shown that people with LBD change their level of consciousness from alert to almost comatose within a matter of seconds. However, the symptoms people observe are that the person will be clear as a bell and alert on one day and then become extremely confused and difficult to arouse, or drowsy, the next day.

Early LBD symptoms affecting memory include difficulty with attention or concentration, due to Lewy bodies in the frontal lobe, and difficulty with short-term memory, due to Lewy bodies in the hippocampus. The attention and concentration difficulties are more severe than the short-term memory loss.

The disease first affects the frontal, parietal, and occipital lobes, all of which can be seen with a SPECT or positron emission tomography (PET, a cousin to SPECT) brain scan early on. Only later, after neurons die off, can an MRI detect atrophy in these brain areas.

Adrienne ✳ A Case of LBD

When Dr. Shankle first saw Adrienne, she had been experiencing symptoms for two years and had already been diagnosed by another neurologist as having Alzheimer's disease. She was taking Aricept, but it wasn't helping her. Her first symptoms included visual hallucinations of dwarf-like friendly people whom she could talk to, a loss of interest in socializing with her friends, and falling down unexpectedly. Later on, she developed urinary incontinence. Physical examinations showed that Adrienne was so unsteady she required a wheelchair. Her face exhibited little in the way of expression, she rarely spoke, and when she did she mumbled. Adrienne had great difficulty recognizing pictures of simple everyday objects. However, her short-term memory was relatively well preserved.

A brain SPECT study was ordered; it showed markedly reduced activity in the occipital, parietal, and frontal lobes. It was clear that Adrienne had LBD. Dr. Shankle started her on a different memory-enhancing med-

Figure 3.4. Adrienne's SPECT Study

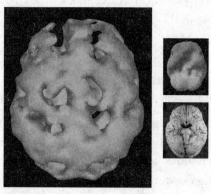

Top view
Reduced occipital, parietal,
and frontal lobe activity

ication, Exelon, which is more helpful in LBD. At her three-month visit, she walked into Dr. Shankle's office and reported in a clear voice that she had regained bladder control and was no longer hallucinating. She also demonstrated her improved speech by giving a detailed (and unsolicited) criticism of Dr. Shankle's attire.

Of all dementing diseases, LBD produces the greatest decline in the neurotransmitter acetylcholine. Consequently, LBD persons often respond dramatically to medications that increase acetylcholine levels. Since both Reminyl and Exelon increase acetylcholine in the brain more than Aricept does, they are likely to produce the best response to LBD.

Parkinson's Disease (PD) and Dementia

Parkinson's disease is caused by loss of neurons that make the neurotransmitter dopamine in a part of the brain that balances muscle movements, such as walking, reaching, grasping, standing, crouching, speaking, and eating.

If you live to the age of 85 and have PD, you have a 2 in 3 chance of becoming demented if you do not reduce its risk factors. The chances of experiencing dementia increase 5 percent for every year the person has PD. In fact, people with PD are from three to six times more likely to develop dementia than those in the general population.

Early Symptoms

Parkinson's disease always starts as a physical movement disorder. The hallmark features of PD are:

- Difficulty starting a movement; a related symptom is reduced eye-blinking, which looks like a stare
- Trouble slowing down movement;
- Muscles feel stiff and resist movement; related symptoms are mumbling (irritates the spouse), leaning to one side, losing balance, and falling
- A rhythmic shaking of the hands or head, when doing nothing (called a resting tremor); it often looks like the person is rolling a pill between the fingers
- Walking with quick, stuttering, small baby steps

Dementia associated with PD always comes later, three or more years after the movement-related symptoms appear.

Diagnosis

A physician diagnosis Parkinson's disease on the basis of a physical exam, a detailed clinical history of the patient, or the presence of the main symptoms.

Joe ❖ Diagnosis of PD Dementia

Joe, who was 73, had had Parkinson's disease for about four years. He managed to play tennis and golf to help minimize the problems he had with coordinating his body movements. In addition, he was an avid reader. Recently, his wife had noticed that he had been looking a lot more confused, that he took longer to respond to questions, that he had begun sleeping in the afternoon, and that on occasion he would fly into a rage for no apparent reason. Joe explained most of it away. He was old, he said, so of course he took a nap during the day. And naturally he got angry once in a while. Who didn't? His wife said it was a change from the way he usually was.

Joe's neurological examination was typical for a person with mild Parkinson's disease. He had mild rigidity in his arms and some delay in starting movements, and when he did move it was a little slow. Joe's mental processes were also slow. His testing showed that he had mild impairment in short-term memory and his processing speed and verbal fluency were slow. His brain SPECT scan showed reduced activity in the basal ganglia. The SPECT scan also showed reduced frontal lobe activity, which caused his working memory and verbal fluency deficits. His SPECT scan and cognitive test results, combined with his symptoms of aggression, confusion, and altered daytime alertness and sleepiness suggested to us that Joe had reduced dopamine and norepinephrine as a result of PD. Therefore, he was started on Wellbutrin, an atypical antidepressant medication that increases dopamine and norepinephrine neurotransmitter activity. After several dose adjustments, Joe's aggression, confusion, and daytime drowsiness disappeared within a few months. He was finally able to resume his favorite pastimes.

Frontal-Temporal Lobe Dementia (FTLD)

This condition, as its name implies, is a series of diseases that affect the frontal lobes and temporal lobes. These disorders are also associated with damage to deep areas of the brain (also called subcortical), including the basal ganglia (which control movements), and the hypothalamus (which regulates hormone release into the bloodstream to regulate the body's organs).

This condition accounts for 10 percent of all cases of dementia and often begins in people who are under 65. This stands in contrast to AD, where people usually first experience symptoms after age 60 (except for rare, early-onset genetic forms of AD). FTLD usually causes progressive and irreversible decline in a person's abilities during a period of two to fifteen years.

The most common causes of FTLD involve abnormalities of the tau protein, the structural backbone of the neuron. Mutations of a gene on chromosome 17 have been found to cause the tau protein to twist into a spiral staircase, blocking the flow of molecules from the cell body to the axon, dendrites, and synapses. This neuronal traffic jam starves the outer reaches of the neuron and causes it to pull its processes in to survive. Eventually, even this attempt to compensate fails, and the neuron dies as a tangled mass of twisted tau proteins, appropriately called a neurofibrillary tangle.

The FTLD diseases produce overlapping symptom groups that fall into four syndromes.

1. *Frontal lobe dementia:* uninhibited behavior with virtually no insight about how if affects others (social disinhibition), apathy, and lack of interest in or disengagement from activities that used to be enjoyable
2. *Primary progressive aphasia:* mainly affects the left temporal lobe and there is a progressive loss of language, beginning about two years before the dementia symptoms develop
3. *Corticobasal degeneration syndrome:* the inability to perform complex tasks, paralysis of voluntary eye movements, lightning-like muscle jerks in response to various stimuli such as bright lights or loud noises, and a failure to recognize a part of one's own body
4. *Amyotrophic lateral sclerosis* (ALS, or Lou Gehrig's disease): spontaneous twitching of specific muscles at rest followed by a wasting away of these muscles, difficulties with swallowing, difficulty speaking or a change in voice pitch, and respiratory distress

Figure 3.5. Typical FTLD SPECT Study

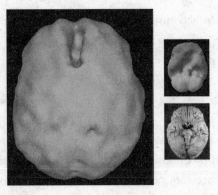

Top view

Early Symptoms

Common early symptoms of FTLD are as follows:

Apathy: A person who is apathetic shows a complete and inexplicable lack of interest in life's little details and pleasures. Because no pleasure is taken in the usual activities, there is a drop in motivation to accomplish anything.

Social disinhibition: This feature is also seen most frequently in the early stages of this disease. It involves the loss of the normal social inhibitions we all take for granted, like not taking one's clothes off in public or not saying exactly what one thinks. It is the result of damage to the underside of the frontal lobes. One of our patients had been a devout Christian his entire life. His wife reported that he had begun trying to have sex with every single female he encountered, including complete strangers, children, little babies, and even female dogs. Another patient, who was a police officer, was referred to us because he had been picked up for brazen shoplifting. Another patient, who had been a senior executive in a prominent Los Angeles law firm, told his wife one day that he had decided to hitchhike across the United States, and with that pronouncement, he walked out the door. He was found weeks later somewhere in Kansas.

Aphasia: This term refers to a sudden inability to understand or use language. This is most frequently seen in primary progressive aphasia. The loss of language skills points to damage to the left temporal lobe. The most frequent problems to be noted early on are either a marked reduction in the amount a person talks or a loss in the spontaneity of her speech during a conversation. We have heard many spouses complain that their partner no longer responds to them, and seems simply uninterested in conversations. Sometimes speech becomes simplified because the person cannot recall the right word. She will say something like "that thing you tell time with" when she means a clock. The naming problem indicates damage to the left tip of the temporal lobe.

Apraxia: This term refers to an inability to perform complex tasks. It is most frequently seen in corticobasal degeneration syndrome and frontal lobe dementia. The problem points to frontal lobe dysfunction in selecting and executing the proper sequence of movements when trying to complete an action or a job; it can range from something as simple as opening a door to something as complex as figure skating. One of Dr. Shankle's patients used to enjoy building model ships, but he began to have trouble assembling the pieces properly. Another patient who was a famous architect began to design buildings that were impossible to construct. His designs resembled an abstract painting more than a real blueprint.

Alien hand syndrome: This is a strange condition in which the person does not recognize a particular part of his body as his own. When we show the patient his arm and say "Does this arm belong to you?" he says no. It is most frequently seen early on in corticobasal degeneration syndrome.

Stereotypical behaviors: Stereotypical behaviors are senseless, repetitive actions or use of language. This is most frequently seen early on in corticobasal degeneration syndrome. Examples of this behavior are excessive clearing of the throat, smiling, frowning, buttoning a shirt, waving goodbye, shaking someone's hand, and reaching for an object. When there is damage to the basal ganglia early on, these behaviors are enacted out of context because they are disconnected from the frontal lobe, meaning the behavior is not supervised by the "executive director." These patients will keep trying to rebutton a buttoned shirt, screw more than one lid onto the same container, continue reaching for an object that is no longer there, stuff objects into their mouths that aren't food, or constantly clear the throat even if nothing is stuck in there.

Paula ❖ *Early Stages of Apathetic Frontal Lobe Dementia*

Paula was a 59-year-old woman who had been actively engaged in church activities as well as in her husband's career. However, her husband indicated that lately she had given up a number of church social activities, and she no longer seemed excited about traveling with him on business. Paula knew of his concerns, but she herself was unconcerned about the changes and didn't understand what the fuss was all about (apathy, lack of interest, disengagement). She explained that as she grew older, she simply wasn't interested in the same things anymore (impaired insight). Her testing showed normal short-term memory and a normal ability to draw complex figures, but it also revealed a mild reduction in the number of words that she could generate, beginning with the letters F, A, and S (according to re-

Figure 3.6. Paula's SPECT Study

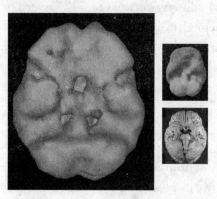

Underside view
Reduced frontal and temporal lobe activity

search this is a sign of damage to the underside of the left frontal lobe). In addition, when she recalled words from a list, she could not remember the sequence in the right order (a sign of impaired working memory as a result of prefrontal damage). When her blood testing and brain MRI came back entirely normal, a brain SPECT scan was ordered, which showed mildly reduced activity in the frontal and temporal lobes.

With treatment over the past eight years, Paula has shown very little deterioration in functioning. In fact, her working memory actually improved with Ritalin, a medication often used for people with attention deficit disorder (ADD). More recently, she has begun to show some impairment in her short-term memory, indicating that the disease has progressed to the hippocampus. However, her short-term memory improved by treatment with Aricept, a medication designed to help with cognitive impairment. Although there is no cure for FTLD, proper treatment can help maintain a good quality of life for years.

For many families, the most devastating aspect of FTLD is often the individual's lack of insight. Persons with FTLD simply do not see themselves as impaired and cannot be reasoned with when they make reckless decisions. This is one situation where preventive action early on can literally save families their entire life savings. Eldercare attorneys specialize in establishing a legal conservator to keep FTLD persons from bringing financial ruin on themselves and their loved ones. Contact your local bar association for attorneys who specialize in eldercare.

The course of FTLD is usually progressive deterioration over two to fifteen years, with most living between six and twelve years.

Vascular Dementia (VD)

This is a syndrome of insufficient blood flow to brain areas that causes cognitive problems. It can be caused by many diseases, the most common being hypertension, diabetes, heart disease, stroke, tobacco smoking, excessive alcohol, and a sedentary lifestyle. VD is a very common type of dementia, which usually begins at age 50 and accounts for 15 to 25 percent of all cases of dementia. It can develop suddenly or gradually, taking as long as 40 years. How quickly it develops depends largely on the severity of the underlying diseases causing it.

Although VD is not hereditary per se, many of the risk factors for it are, so VD does tend to run in families. It can result from a single large stroke or hemorrhage in the brain or from an accumulation of many smaller strokes or hemorrhages. The common mechanism for all types of VD is:

1. Blood vessels fail to deliver blood containing oxygen and glucose to brain cells
2. Within minutes brain cells are damaged by the loss of these essential nutrients
3. Brain cells die if blood flow is not restored quickly

When a large blood vessel fails to deliver blood to brain cells, a major disability suddenly occurs. Large strokes are familiar because they are easily observable and are usually treated in hospital emergency rooms. However, large strokes are not the most common cause of VD. The accumulation of small strokes that go unrecognized for years is more common. According to the National Stroke Association, VD is largely preventable by directly treating the major stroke risk factors, which are:

- Poorly controlled hypertension
- Diabetes (causes blood vessels to become brittle and to break more easily)
- Atherosclerosis (hardening of the arteries of the brain or heart, often with high cholesterol)
- Heart diseases that produce blood clots or reduce blood flow to the brain, including congestive heart failure, coronary artery disease, heart attack, and irregular heart rhythms
- Coronary artery bypass surgery, which can be avoided by treating coronary artery disease
- Smoking (constricts blood vessels and decreases blood flow)
- Excessive caffeine use (also constricts blood vessels and decreases blood flow)
- Amphetamine or cocaine drug use (constricts blood vessels and causes hemorrhages)
- Heavy alcohol use (more than four glasses of wine or the equivalent in hard liquor daily accounts for about 5 percent of all strokes)
- Narrowing of the blood vessels in the neck, which delivers blood to the front of the brain
- Transient ischemic attacks, which are strokes that resolve themselves within 24 hours
- Previous stroke (165,000 people in the United States die of stroke each year, making it the third leading cause of death, with heart disease and cancer in the lead, and AD fourth)
- Elevated levels of the amino acid homocysteine, which also increases the risk for AD

Subcortical Vascular Dementia (SVD)

SVD is the most common type of vascular dementia. It affects the small blood vessels that deliver blood to the brain areas below the cortex (hence the name subcortical). The onset of SVD usually occurs after age 50. It is gradually progressive, and often the person is unaware of any problems for years. One of the tricky and misleading things about SVD is that a problem does not consistently occur. Sometimes a person will not remember a conversation or recent place visited, while at other times memory is fine. This inconsistent difficulty represents a distinct change in the person's previous abilities.

The blood supply to the subcortical areas comes from the blood vessels at the brain's surface, which branch off and dive down like straight plumbing pipes. The subcortical areas are the farthest from the heart of any place in the brain and become starved of glucose and oxygen when any of the following occurs:

- The pipe-like vessels become narrow, rigid or clogged
- The heart just doesn't pump forcefully enough
- The blood thickens or clots too easily

Under these conditions, literally thousands of small strokes will accumulate over years. Rarely will any of these small strokes cause symptoms, but as they accumulate over time, there will be a gradual development of symptoms related to the functions of the areas affected.

Coronary Bypass Graft Surgery and SVD

When the coronary arteries narrow and can no longer deliver blood to the heart muscle, strokes in the heart occur. These are commonly known as heart attacks. Coronary artery bypass graft surgery (CABG) is an effective operation that bypasses these clogged coronary arteries and delivers blood to the heart muscle to prevent heart attacks. Worldwide, 800,000 patients undergo CABG surgery each year, and in the United States, 500,000. Stroke, cognitive impairment, and confusion are common complications that result from clots or debris released during this surgery, and they can occur for up to three months after the surgery.

Until recently, CABG surgery was not thought to be a cause of dementia. However, a study of CABG surgery patients that followed them for five years after surgery showed that their risk of SVD progressively increased (31). This increased risk was independent of other VD risk factors typically found in persons undergoing CABG surgery (age, hypertension, diabetes, stroke, heart disease, and so on). It is not known whether CABG surgery patients with good blood flow from the heart are less likely to develop SVD than those with relatively poorer blood flow from the heart. If heart muscle strength turns out to explain the risk associated with CABG surgery, then measuring both cognitive function and cardiac output (the pump force of the heart muscle) before and after surgery, as well as annually thereafter, will help prevent SVD by allowing the physician to know when to intervene. Other VD risk factors must, of course, be minimized.

Early Symptoms

There are three main early symptoms of subcortical VD, as follows.

1. *Impaired task performance.* Because fuel is cut off from white matter deep in the brain, the breakdown of complex skills can manifest in many ways:

- Impaired attention
- Apathy
- Impaired judgment
- Mental slowing down or taking longer to perform the same task
- Difficulty shifting from one part of a task to the next
- Performing the task at a lower level of expertise or in a simpler way
- Difficulty expressing words or doing tasks

2. *Walking problems.* The deepest white matter fibers also control leg movements, so these are often among the early symptoms. Walking may either be slow or clumsy.

3. *Clumsiness.* Inaccurate and uncoordinated movements can occur when writing, putting dishes away, inserting a key into a lock, brushing teeth, doing fine needlework, and so on.

Diagnosis

The two key aspects of diagnosis are the presence of cognitive impairment and evidence of stroke or hemorrhage. Alzheimer's disease and VD share many of the same risk factors, and many who have AD also have VD. Consequently, a diagnosis of VD should be made independently of AD, so both can be diagnosed and treated. In general, a diagnosis of VD should not be made unless strokes are seen on an MRI. Other supportive evidence includes neurological signs detected by the examining physician and an irregular course of sudden changes in function followed by partial improvement and then followed by periods of little to no change. However, there may be no neurological signs, and the course may have been gradual.

Mark ❖ Early Vascular Dementia

Mark was a 58-year-old man with a high-pressure sales job that required him to entertain his clients a great deal. He had a history of hypertension that would "get a little high" at times, and diabetes that he thought was "diet-controlled." His cholesterol was in the 250s. Over the past year, his wife noticed that he would sometimes forget to take his high-blood-pressure medication, had become far less talkative, occasionally lost his balance for no apparent reason, and would sometimes grow inappropriately aggressive toward her and others.

When Mark was seen by Dr. Shankle he explained that his problems were caused by more pressure at work than usual and that he would be fine. However, upon neurological examination, Mark showed a slight weakness in his right arm, and the right side of his mouth drooped slightly. His eyes also jerked involuntarily when he looked to one side. Mark's neuropsychological testing showed that he often made careless mistakes, had a shortened attention span (working memory), and had some trouble with naming objects he did not use a lot, like a tripod. His MRI showed that strokes had affected the subcortical areas of his brain, particularly on the left side.

Mark's treatment involved correcting his blood pressure and diabetes first, by first making sure he took his medication. To do this, his wife had to supervise his medications, checking that he faithfully took them day and night. A trial of the acetylcholinesterase inhibitor Reminyl created significant improvement in his working memory and attention span. His temper improved, and for over a year now he has remained stable. If the underlying risk factors for VD can be controlled, then the dementia can often be stopped and sometimes reversed, at least partially. This is particularly true if the diagnosis of VD is made early on.

Cancers and Cancer Treatments That Can Cause Dementia

Cancer can start in any organ or tissue in your body, and can spread through the bloodstream and lymph glands. Cancers of the lung, breast, kidney, liver, heart, prostate, gut, skin, bone, and blood are the most likely to spread to the brain and cause cognitive impairment or dementia. In the future, we are likely to see more cancer cures from treatment advances. But there may be a cost. Cognitive impairment and dementia are increasingly recognized as long-term complications of cancer therapy. Most cancer treatments, such as chemotherapy and radiation therapy, kill not only cancer cells but also normal cells. This means that when the treatment affects brain cells, part of the brain is being destroyed to save the patient's life. Radiation therapy is sometimes given to the brain to either prevent or to treat brain cancers, and this does direct damage to the brain. Many cancer chemotherapy medications go straight to the brain, and they target not only dividing cancer cells but also any normal brain cells that are dividing. While the problem area is targeted and destroyed, there are always "innocent bystanders" caught in the crossfire.

Early Symptoms

Cognitive impairment due to cancer and its treatments is still a poorly studied area, because until recently, most cancer patients did not live long enough to develop these problems. The specific type of cognitive impairment that develops depends on where the cancer cells reside in the brain. When radiation therapy includes the brain, the primary areas damaged are the deep areas of the brain, so the symptoms that develop resemble VD and FTLD. The cognitive impairment produced by radiation therapy can be long-lasting. For example, a study of patients who had received radiation therapy to the sinuses up to 20 years prior found impairments of working memory, eye-hand coordination, manual dexterity, and judgment.

Dementia Due to Head Injury

Brain trauma from head injury is more common in the United States than most people realize, with two million new cases a year being reported. Brain trauma can cause dementia or make it worse. It is particularly dangerous in the 15 to 25 percent of the population who have the apolipoprotein E4 gene, the genetic factor that increases risk for Alzheimer's disease. If people with this gene also happen to experience a loss of consciousness from a head injury, their risk of developing AD increases tenfold (32)! In people who do not have the apolipoprotein E4 gene, the risk of developing AD after a head injury does not increase. Consider the fact that during the career of virtually every professional football, hockey, basketball, and soccer player, they have had at least one head injury and lost consciousness. This means that 15 to 25 percent of these athletes are about 10 times more likely to develop Alzheimer's disease. It also means that 300,000 to 500,000 of the 2 million new cases of brain trauma each year are ten times more likely to develop AD. These are frightening statistics.

Head injury damages the brain in several ways.

1. At the site of impact, the blood vessels may tear and cause bleeding, inflammation, and scarring. This disrupted blood supply can impede the removal of free radicals that are released by the damaged cells, which then causes further tissue damage.
2. The impact accelerates the brain to ram into the opposite end of the skull to produce a second site of damage, called a contra-coup injury. Years later, a SPECT scan on such a person may show a loss of brain activity in both places.
3. The accelerating brain shears and tears the axons, which disrupts the brain's long-distance communication cables. The brain's repair system tries to reconnect these severed cables by creating "guide wires" out of supportive brain cells; sometimes it succeeds. However, if the guide wires do not accurately line up the cut ends of the axons, they will not reconnect. In this case, communication between the disconnected brain areas either slows down or fails altogether.

Dr. Amen's SPECT brain imaging work has shown that even mild head injuries with brief periods of unconsciousness (seconds to minutes)—the kind of trauma that people routinely shake off as unimportant—can be more damaging than most physicians realize. While brain computerized tomography (CT) and MRI scans reveal the most severe consequences of brain damage, such as hemorrhage or tissue loss, brain SPECT and PET scans show much subtler and more widespread changes.

Head injury can also unmask Alzheimer's disease. We have seen many patients whose families first recognized signs of memory loss in a loved one after a mild head injury occurred. When examined, however, these patients often have other cognitive impairments that cannot be explained by the head injury alone. Their Alzheimer's disease had previously gone undetected because the symptoms were too subtle to notice.

Because of the nature and structure of the brain, even mild head injuries should be treated. Your brain can be damaged even without the loss of consciousness. One only loses consciousness when the brain stem is damaged or when both sides of the brain are injured. It is quite possible for the rest of the brain, which is equally vulnerable, to sustain significant trauma from injuries without losing consciousness.

Early Symptoms

Three groups of early symptoms occur with cognitive impairment due to head injury

1. *Symptoms due to injuring the brain areas affected by the impact and contracoup sites.* For example, a person gets in a car accident and hits her head against the windshield, producing frontal (impact site) and occipital (contracoup site) lobe damage. She could feel apathetic, have changes in her vision, and have difficulty concentrating.

2. *Symptoms due to diffuse axonal injury.* These include slowing of mental abilities, such as taking longer to think of someone's name, to add numbers, or to fit a key into a lock.

3. *Symptoms due to damaging brain areas that rest on the base of the skull,* which are the undersides of the frontal and temporal lobes, the cerebellum,

the pituitary, and hypothalamus. When the head injury accelerates the brain, these areas are abraded. Common symptoms include clumsiness, difficulty recognizing faces and objects, short-term memory loss, inappropriate aggressive or impulsive behavior, loss of energy, disturbed sleep, and daytime drowsiness.

Diagnosis

Obviously, knowing that the patient has had a head injury in the past is essential for accurate diagnosis. Many people, however, forget the head injuries they have been exposed to, especially when they were children. For patients who come to our clinics, it is not uncommon to have to ask them five times whether or not they have had a head injury before they think back carefully enough to remember one.

Bill ❖

By the time Bill sought help, he was 65. He was depressed, suicidal, and lethargic, and he had a very short attention span. All his life he had struggled with a short fuse, and he had lost several wives and alienated his children because of it. He and his girlfriend of two years had just broken up because of his temper. When asking about his history, it was discovered that he had been in a car accident when in high school. He was with a friend who had been drinking. The friend lost control of the car one night, and Bill did not have his seat belt on. His head cracked the windshield of the car; he did not remember whether or not he lost consciousness. At that time, he was between grades—tenth and eleventh. Before the accident, he had done very well in school, but in the semester following it, he did so poorly that he gave up his dream of going to a top-rung university. "I couldn't pay attention anymore," he said. "My mind was always wandering off the task at hand." After high school, Bill had gone to work for his father's business. So he had job security but not peace of mind—he and his father fought constantly over Bill's behavior. Bill frequently lost interest, took time off work, and didn't finish tasks that were assigned to him.

A SPECT study was ordered to evaluate Bill's underlying brain metabolism. It was significantly abnormal. He had serious decreased activity of the frontal and temporal lobes. Seeing the scan was extremely helpful

Figure 3.7. Bill's Rest and Concentration SPECT Series

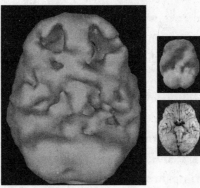

Underside view
Decreased prefrontal and
temporal lobe activity

for Bill, because it made him feel that he finally had an explanation for why he had had to struggle all those years. He was also hopeful for the first time that he could do something to help himself. With a combination of anticonvulsant and stimulant medication, as well as a special treatment called neurofeedback, which helps to stabilize electrical activity over the left prefrontal and temporal lobe regions, his mood, temper, and attention span were able to stabilize. Once Bill's girlfriend realized his problems were the consequence of a medical problem that he was dealing with (as opposed to the idea that he was just a difficult person), she came back to him.

Depending on what brain areas are affected, head injury can produce different types of impairments. And the treatment depends on which brain systems are involved, which can be clearly identified with SPECT or PET imaging. The best treatment, however, is prevention. Our imaging work has taught us time and again how devastating head injuries can be and how dangerous head contact sports are, particularly for those who are already at risk for Alzheimer's disease. When your child wants to sign up for soccer, football, rugby, or other sports that pose a significant risk for trauma to the skull, take him to the driving range or the tennis court.

Infectious and Immunological Causes of Dementia

If any number of infectious organisms—including prions, viruses, bacteria, and fungi—invade the brain and the infection is not stopped either by the immune system or medication, dementia can occur. Infectious agents can enter the cell, insert themselves somewhere into the cell's machinery, and then take control. From there they replicate and repeat the process, taking over more and more cells. Normally, the immune system will eliminate most infections and other agents that are foreign to the body. But when the immune system is not working properly or is overwhelmed by infection, cognitive impairment or dementia can occur.

Sometimes the infection is not the only cause of the dementia but adds to an underlying problem. Many families have said that after their loved one developed pneumonia, he or she began to be confused, and the condition didn't go away when the illness resolved. Such individuals may have already had Alzheimer's disease or some other cause of dementia, but it was too mild to be detected by casual observation. The most common types of infection or immune dysfunction that can cause cognitive impairment or dementia include:

- Multiple sclerosis (MS), which damages the insulation (myelin) of the nerve fibers in the brain and causes a wide variety of neurological problems
- Chronic fatigue immunodeficiency syndrome (CFIDS)
- Creutzfeld-Jakob disease (CJD), or "mad cow disease"
- Herpes viruses (herpes simplex), Cytomegalovirus (CMV), Varicella-Zoster, also known as chicken pox or shingles (VZ), Epstein-Barr virus (EBV), and human herpes 6 (HH6)
- Human immunodeficiency viruses (HIV), which can lead to acquired immune deficiency syndrome (AIDS), which predispose individuals to a great many types of infections that can invade the brain
- Bacterial infections of the heart or brain

We will explore CFIDS in more detail because it is commonly misunderstood and is often an incorrectly treated cause of dementia.

Chronic Fatigue Immunodeficiency Syndrome (CFIDS)

This term refers to a combination of immune deficiency plus infection by any of a number of infectious agents that are normally destroyed by the immune system. The common viruses that attack CFIDS patients are EBV, CMV, and HH6. Unfortunately many doctors believe CFIDS patients only have psychological problems and that CFIDS is not a "real" disease. These doctors are wrong. In fact, just recently it was shown that EBV, one of the viruses commonly found in CFIDS, is found in persons an average of four years before they come down with multiple sclerosis! It should be understood that CFIDS is a very real disease (or collection of diseases), and there are objective ways of diagnosing the immune deficiency that gives rise to the ensuing problems. The patterns of symptoms are quite consistent among individuals, and they cannot be explained away purely by depression, anxiety, or other psychological symptoms.

Early Symptoms

Patients who develop CFIDS often describe the first signs of it as a bad cold or the flu. While other people usually get over the flu or cold, these patients often develop severe bouts of fatigue, numbness and tingling in their arms and legs, generalized body aches, and difficulty concentrating. These bouts can come and go for years. Sometimes CFIDS disappears spontaneously; at others it continues, severely curtailing people's lives. Such patients do develop psychological symptoms like depression, low self-esteem, apathy, and anxiety. Indeed, it would be surprising, given the unrelenting physical illnesses that episodically disable them without warning, if they did not experience emotional repercussions.

This syndrome can damage any part of the brain but particularly targets the temporal lobes. Temporal lobe seizures can add to a CFIDS person's cognitive impairment. Temporal lobe seizures bring on a sudden onset of bizarre symptoms like confusion, an inability to speak or comprehend what is being said, flashbacks, déjà vu, intense paranoia or fear for no good reason, and more. A number of famous artists, such as Gauguin and Van Gogh, had temporal lobe seizures, which, while debilitating, may have also been, in part at least, a source of inspiration or creativity.

Diagnosis

An accurate report of early symptoms helps in diagnosing CFIDS. In addition, an immunological evaluation of the blood is quite useful. Most physicians are not experts at evaluating CFIDS, so an infectious disease specialist, immunologist, or CFIDS specialist should be consulted to make sure the diagnosis is correct. Ask your family physician for a referral to one of these specialists.

Brain SPECT scans of CFIDS persons often show severe overall reduced activity, especially in the frontal and temporal lobes, which is similar to what appears in FTLD or diffuse toxic exposure. But the exact pattern that is present depends to some degree on which viruses are present, because they each have their own favorite part of the brain to inhabit. The principal value of SPECT in diagnosing CFIDS is its ability to identify which brain systems are most involved. This knowledge helps guide the treatment and avoid costly financial and personal wrong turns on the path to health.

Denise ✤ CFIDS

Denise, 45 years old, was a mother of two who had been active all her life. She was a devoted mother, worked with her husband in their business every day, and served on the boards of a number of charities. Several years prior to consulting with us she had come down with the flu; it took almost a month to get better. About two months after that, she developed a case of fatigue so intense that she could not get out of bed for days at a time. She reported that she also experienced "cloudy thinking," a loss of motivation to do almost anything, and numbness and tingling in her hands and feet. Occasionally her symptoms would clear up, but never entirely. She did the best she could to keep up with her activities, but when these episodes occurred, she was so disabled that she had trouble taking care of her children. Another complication was that she had recently begun experiencing a sudden onset of intense confusion and fear, which would last for a few minutes and then go away (temporal lobe seizures).

Denise had already been to several psychiatrists, who treated her for depression, apathy, and hypothyroidism. While these treatments helped to some degree, the disabling episodes continued unabated. When Dr. Shankle first saw her she had a normal neurological examination. Her neuropsychologic testing illustrated mild impairment for a woman her age and education as well as left interior frontal lobe damage.

The combination of an impaired working memory and flu-like illness followed by physical and psychological symptoms led to a referral to an immunologist for an evaluation for possible immune deficiency. Her blood testing showed that her killer T-cells (immune cells that recognize foreign bodies like infectious organisms and then destroy them) did not function well. She also had a number of viruses (EBV, CMV and HH6), which would be suppressed by a healthy person's immune system. There was no question that Denise had CFIDS.

Her SPECT scan showed that she had reduced overall activity, especially in the frontal lobes and temporal lobes. Because of her symptoms, she was treated with a small dose of Trileptal, which is an anticonvulsant that can treat temporal lobe seizures while still minimizing the chance of producing cognitive impairment, and Adderall, a medication that increases energy and working memory. In addition, she continued to see the immunologist to give her gamma globulin infusions to reduce the chance

Figure 3.8. Denise's SPECT Study

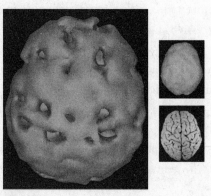

Top view
Decreased activity in many
brain areas

of bouts of fatigue and other symptoms. The gamma globulin minimized the frequency and the severity of the fatigue episodes. The Adderall significantly helped her during her bouts of fatigue, and most of the time it improved her ability to focus and concentrate. She no longer has temporal lobe seizures.

Although CFIDS is not curable, the impact it has on the patient's life can be greatly alleviated with proper treatment.

Alcohol-Related Dementia and Other Brain Toxins

Many toxins attack brain function and cause dementia, and each one has its own way of damaging the brain. Some of the more common toxins or medications that can harm the brain are:

- Addictive drugs, such as tranquilizers, sedatives, cocaine, speed, LSD, and others
- Alcohol
- Anticonvulsants (seizure medications)
- Toxic fumes, pesticides, and other industrial chemicals

Alcohol-Related Dementia

By far the most common toxin that causes dementia in this country is alcohol, ingested in excessive amounts. Alcohol affects the brain profoundly by

- Blocking the entry of calcium into cells to inhibit neurotransmitter release and reduce the neuron's electrical activity
- Blocking the transport of oxygen into the cell's energy-production centers
- Reducing the effectiveness of many different types of neurotransmitters, especially those involved in learning and remembering

Alcohol is a double-edged sword; depending on the quantity of intake, it can either help or injure a person's health. Large amounts of it—four or more glasses of wine, or the equivalent in hard liquor—on a daily basis, increase the risk of vascular dementia. However, it has been found that small amounts—a glass of wine once a week or once a month but not daily—may *significantly reduce dementia by up to 70 percent* (33). The reduced risk seems to be related to the fact that alcohol and cholesterol compete with each other and sometimes it is good for alcohol to win. Small amounts of alcohol compete with HDL, the good cholesterol, which actually removes the harmful types of cholesterol. When a person drinks a little alcohol, HDL is not allowed to bind to the cell membrane, so it is forced back into the bloodstream, where it lowers LDL and other harmful cholesterols. This reduces the person's risk of heart disease, atherosclerosis, and strokes, all of which are known causes for dementia.

Alcohol problems are often hereditary. Many alcoholics have low levels of the primary inhibitory neurotransmitter of the brain, GABA; GABA neurons play an important role in the functioning of the brain: they enhance function by inhibiting neuronal activity to control the brain's level of excitation. If GABA levels are low, however, as they are in people susceptible to alcoholism, then the activity is not inhibited as much as it should be. The brain grows too excited, and this is often experienced as anxiety, agitation, nervousness, frustration, or hyperactivity. The person then drinks alcohol because it temporarily lowers the anxiety, but the price of drinking alcohol on a daily basis is very high.

Withdrawal time from alcohol is relatively short (less than two weeks), but treating alcohol-related dementia is a good deal more difficult. The constant use of alcohol makes the brain unresponsive to its own neurotransmitters, causing something like a generalized power failure. When cognitive impairment or dementia sets in, it is frequently in the form of being unable to understand why it is in one's own best interest to stop drinking alcohol. One has lost one's insight and cannot be reasoned with to stop drinking. Many simply do not see or acknowledge that they even have a serious condition. Compounding the problem, alcohol has made the brain resistant to whatever beneficial effects could be received from most medications or behavioral therapies, so that large amounts may be needed.

The loss of insight can be profound. One patient of Dr. Shankle's repeatedly accused his daughter of interfering with his life. He said that he would only have one vodka martini after dinner and was not an alcoholic. His daughter indicated he would drink four or more martinis each night and would forget each one he drank. Evaluation showed that he had dementia due to alcohol abuse. Dr. Shankle showed him objective tests to try and convince him that he had severe memory loss and severely impaired judgment about his own memory ability (he estimated that he would recall nine of ten words after a two-minute delay, and he recalled zero). Dr. Shankle told him that unless he stopped drinking, he would be in a nursing home in six months. His daughter tried many approaches to getting him to stop drinking, but he simply could not be convinced that he had a drinking or memory problem. He now resides in a nursing home.

Early Symptoms

Preoccupation with drinking, hangovers, impaired judgment, thoughtless or risky behavior, clouded thinking, withdrawal anxiety, isolated drinking, defensiveness about drinking, and denial are all common in alcohol abuse. A "blackout" is a later symptom, in which a person wakes up after a bout with alcohol and has no memory whatsoever of a certain time period. This amnesia points to the fact that alcohol damaged the ability of the hippocampus and entorhinal cortex to store new memories during the intoxication. All the hints in the world will not help someone recall what was never stored in the first place. Sedatives and tranquilizers such as Valium, Ativan, Xanax, Serax, Restoril, and Halcion can produce the same effect. Symptoms such as incoordination, unsteadiness, and tremors are associated with alcohol's damage to the cerebellum. Spatial abilities, such as the capacity to draw complex figures or recognize complex patterns, may also be impaired.

Diagnosis

The signs of alcohol abuse are often quite clear because it undermines brain function in many ways. Some people do not drink every day. Instead they binge, which means they drink too much on occasion but do not drink continuously. These people may also sustain alcohol-related brain damage, but to a lesser degree. Early symptoms include clumsiness, balance problems, poor attention and working memory span, and amnesia about recent events. Brain MRI scans show tissue loss, while SPECT and PET scans show reduced activity in the cerebellum, medial temporal lobes, and frontal lobes.

Elsie ✤ Alcohol-Related Dementia

Elsie lived and socialized heavily in Newport Beach, California, for most of her life. She was 70 years old, and for the past 30 years she had drunk at least a quart of scotch a day. Her husband brought her for evaluation because she had become increasingly offensive to their friends during social gatherings. She would make overt sexual advances toward other women's husbands and then have no recollection of her behavior the next day. When she first came to the office, she tried to flirt with Dr. Shankle. She seemed oblivious to why her husband had brought her in and asked Dr. Shankle if he knew why. Within a minute, she forgot that she had asked, and then asked again.

Out of 10 words presented to her, she could recall only one, even after three separate learning trials. After a few minutes went by, she could not even remember that she had ever been asked to recall a list of words. Her spatial abilities were mildly impaired; she had difficulty drawing the internal lines of a cube. Her SPECT scan revealed severe overall reduced activity.

Figures 3.9-10. Elsie's SPECT

Overall severe decreased activity

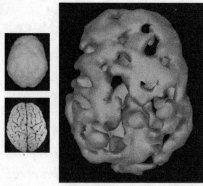 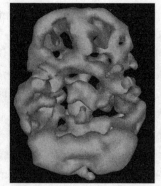 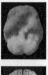 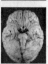

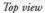 *Top view*   *Underside view*

Elsie was sent to an alcohol treatment program and medically withdrawn from alcohol to prevent delirium tremens (DTs), which can be very dangerous. Vitamins, especially folate, were given, along with a regimen of medicines and supplements to enhance brain function. Even though she never fully regained her faculties, her memory and behavior improved.

If alcoholics are able to quit before too much brain tissue is lost, they can show a marked improvement in their abilities. For reasons we do not yet understand, it often takes up to six months to see the full benefits of stopping drinking.

Disorders Affecting Nerve Cell Metabolism

Virtually every organ is involved in maintaining normal cell metabolism throughout the body. Widespread damage to any of the major organ systems can be toxic to brain cells and result in dementia. Here are common metabolic causes of dementia:

- Depression, due to low levels of neurotransmitters that help cells work efficiently
- Hypothyroidism (low thyroid hormone levels)
- Diabetes (high glucose levels)
- Hypoglycemia (low glucose levels)
- Kidney, liver, or lung failure
- Normal pressure hydrocephalus (excessive production of cerebrospinal fluid)
- Seizures (excessive neuronal excitation)
- Hypoxia (low oxygen levels)
- Low B vitamin levels, including B_{12}, thiamine, or folic acid (can be the result of a number of causes, including alcohol abuse, poor diet, or poor absorption in the stomach)
- High calcium levels, which can be the result of excessive parathyroid hormone activity
- High homocysteine levels, which are regulated by folic acid metabolism
- Low estrogen levels, which occur when hysterectomies are performed after menopause

- Low testosterone levels, which are becoming increasingly recognized in aging men and can sometimes be the result of treatment for prostate cancer
- High or low cortisol levels, which can be the result of chronic stress, a number of diseases, or long-term treatment with corticosteroids such as prednisone

Early Symptoms

The early symptoms of metabolic encephalopathy relate to the impairment of neuronal metabolism, meaning that the mind simply works slower. The patient will take longer to finish her usual tasks, be less attentive, have difficulty concentrating, grow tired easily, or become depressed or apathetic or socially withdrawn.

Diagnosis

The symptoms just described, unfortunately, are all too often dismissed by physicians as the result of "just getting old." We have heard this explanation given to patients by well-meaning doctors who are trying to reassure them that nothing is really wrong with them. However, it should be noted that by the time a patient gets around to mentioning a problem to his doctor, it is usually significant, and it should be taken seriously.

The evaluation for metabolic encephalopathy is fairly straightforward. The first thing to do is to inquire whether there is an underlying medical problem that is getting worse and causing these symptoms. If so, the problem should be treated. Next, a standard set of blood tests can be evaluated for the common causes of metabolic encephalopathy. These tests are discussed in detail in Chapter 7.

Wanda ✦ *"Pseudodementia" of Depression*

Wanda was a 67-year-old woman whose mother had died of Alzheimer's disease. Because Wanda had been her mother's primary caretaker, she had watched her die, and was terrified of the same fate befalling her. For the past two years, she had been noticing quite a bit of difficulty remembering names and recent events. She had also grown very depressed and had withdrawn from society. She was so down that she even had trouble getting

around to daily chores and paying bills. Her family brought her in for evaluation.

Wanda was very aware of her memory loss. Her neurological examination was normal, the results of her cognitive testing were consistent with
depression, and her MRI was entirely normal, revealing no brain tissue loss
in the hippocampus or elsewhere. However, a brain SPECT scan showed
full overall activity, except for decreased activity in her prefrontal cortex at
rest that improved with concentration, and marked increased activity in
her emotional brain, which is a pattern most often seen with depression.

We treated her with an activating antidepressant, Effexor, because she
also experienced apathy. Within three months, Wanda's depression, apathy, and symptoms of memory loss had lifted. We repeated her brain
SPECT scan to see if it had changed as well. It now looked normal, except
for a few small areas of reduced activity.

The cognitive impairment of depression is referred to as pseudodementia because the symptoms can be lifted when the depression is ade-
quately treated. However, this name does injustice to the person suffering
with the symptoms, because there is nothing "pseudo" about his experience of depression and diminished capacity, and because what he is going
through is just as debilitating as other causes of dementia.

The brain is a complex, adaptive system; its goal is to maintain the function of its more than 50 different circuits so that your mind and body can
work together to pursue a satisfying and happy life. Many causes of cognitive impairment or dementia can be treated or improved significantly, if
they are detected early. As we have emphasized, if you wish to take care of
your brain, annual screening for memory loss is just as essential as mam-
mography screening for detecting breast cancer, blood pressure screening
for detecting hypertension, and glucose screening for detecting diabetes.
Once you reach the age of 50, or if you have significant risk factors, you
should have your memory checked on a regular basis.

chapter 4

Know Your Risk: The Shankle-Amen Early Dementia Detection Questionnaire

If there is a family history of dementia, then annual screening after the age of 40 is important. There are actually two purposes for screening at such a young age. First, it is useful to establish a baseline against which various preventive therapies can be measured. Second, establishing a baseline allows earlier detection of any disorders that cause memory loss or dementia, which allows them to be treated in their earliest stage to most effectively prevent or delay their progression.

The Shankle-Amen Early Dementia Detection Questionnaire

The following questionnaire is meant as a general screening tool of cognitive function to indicate whether you should consider further testing. Annual screening is essential to take full advantage of the preventive and disease therapies that are now available and can mean the difference between living your life without the symptoms of Alzheimer's disease and being in a nursing home.

The questionnaire is a two-part self-administered questionnaire that screens for the risk factors associated with ADRD as well as its earliest symptoms. Self-report questionnaires have advantages and limitations. They are quick, inexpensive, and easy to score. On the other hand, people may fill out questionnaires portraying themselves in a way they want to be perceived, resulting in self-report bias. For example, some people exaggerate their experience and mark all of the symptoms as a frequent problem, in essence saying, "I'm glad to have a problem so that I can get help, be sick, or have an excuse for the problems I have." Others are in total denial. They do not want to see any personal flaws and they do not check any symptoms as problematic, in essence saying, "I'm okay. There's nothing wrong with me. Leave me alone."

Not all self-report bias is intentional. People may genuinely have difficulty recognizing problems and expressing how they feel. Right-hemisphere brain problems are classically associated with denial. Sometimes family members or friends are better at evaluating a loved one's level of functioning than a person evaluating himself. They may have noticed things that their loved one hasn't. We believe that you should fill out the questionnaire for yourself and have another person who knows you well also fill it out.

Questionnaires of any sort should never be used alone as an assessment tool. Like an isolated laboratory test result, they are not meant to provide a diagnosis. They are simply catalysts to initiate the process of further evaluation. This questionnaire is a useful first step to help determine whether you or a loved one should do annual screening. In Appendix A, you will find more information on Dr. Shankle's online Memory Screen, Depression Screen, and Mental Skills Test, should you wish to explore your risk further.

The Shankle-Amen Early Dementia Detection Questionnaire

Please answer the following questions with a yes or no. For every yes answer a score is provided parenthetically; add your score at the end of the test for your interpretation. To give yourself the most complete picture, have another person who knows you well also answer the questions (such as a spouse, lover, child, sibling, parent, or close friend or colleague).

1. _NO_ (3.5) One family member with Alzheimer's disease or other cause of dementia
2. _NO_ (7.5) More than one family member with Alzheimer's disease or other dementia
3. _NO_ (2.7) Family history of Down syndrome
4. _YOU_ (2.0) A single head injury with loss of consciousness for more than a few minutes
5. _Yes_ (2.0) Several head injuries without loss of consciousness
6. _Yes_ (4.4) Alcohol dependence or drug dependence in past or present
7. _Yes_ (2.0) Major depression diagnosed by a physician in past or present
8. _No_ (10) Stroke
9. _NO_ (2.5) Heart (coronary artery) disease or heart attack (myocardial infarction, or MI)
10. _NO_ (2.1) High cholesterol (hyperlipidemia)
11. _NO_ (2.3) High blood pressure (hypertension)
12. _NO_ (3.4) Diabetes
13. _Yes_ (3.0) History of cancer or cancer treatment
14. _No_ (1.5) Seizures in past or present
15. _No_ (2.0) Limited exercise (less than twice a week or less than 30 minutes per session)
16. _No_ (2.0) Less than a high school education
17. _No_ (2.0) Jobs that do not require periodically learning new information
18. _Yes_ (2.0) Within the age range 65 to 74 years old
19. _NO_ (7.0) Within the age range 75 to 84 years old
20. _No_ (38.0) Over 85 years old
21. _Yes_ (2.3) Smoking cigarettes for 10 years or longer

(continued)

22. _____ (2.5) Has one apolipoprotein E4 gene (if known)
23. _____ (5.0) Has two apolipoprotein E4 genes (if known)

_____ **Total Score** (Add up the scores in parentheses for all items checked)

Interpretation

If the score is 0, 1, or 2, then you have low risk factors for developing ADRD.

If the score is 3, 4, 5 or 6, then you should annually screen (see Appendix A) after age 50.

If the score is greater than 6, then you should annually screen (see Appendix A) after age 40.

Severity	Progression	Brain Area Involved
Yes, present now	A lot worse than 10 years ago	**TEMPORAL LOBE QUESTIONS**
✓		Is there frequent difficulty remembering appointments?
		Is there frequent difficulty remembering holidays or special occasions such as birthdays or weddings?
		Is there frequent difficulty remembering to take medications or supplements?
		Is there frequent difficulty finding the right words during conversations or retrieving the names of things?
✓		Are there frequent episodes of irritability, anger, aggression, or a "short fuse" for little or no reason?
		Are there frequent episodes of suspiciousness, paranoia, or hypersensitivity without a clear explanation or reason why?
		Is there a frequent tendency to misinterpret what one hears, reads, or experiences?
		Temporal Lobe Severity and Progression Totals (add up the total number of checks for this section in each column)

Severity	Progression	
Yes, present now	**A lot worse than 10 years ago**	**FRONTAL LOBE QUESTIONS**
		Is there frequent difficulty recalling events that occurred a long time ago?
		Is there frequent difficulty with judgments, such as knowing how much food to buy?
		Is there frequent difficulty thinking things through (reasoning)?
		Is there frequent difficulty handling finances or routine affairs that used to be done without difficulty?
√		Is there frequent trouble sustaining attention in routine situations (e.g., chores, paperwork)?
√		Is there frequent difficulty finishing chores, tasks, or other activities?
		Is there frequent difficulty with organizing and planning things?
√		Are there frequent feelings of boredom, loss of interest, or low motivation to do things that were previously enjoyed?
		Is there a frequent tendency to act impulsively, such as saying or doing things without thinking first?
		Frontal Lobe Progression and Severity Totals (add up the total number of checks for this section in each column)
Severity	**Progression**	
Yes, present now	**A lot worse than 10 years ago**	**PARIETAL LOBE QUESTIONS**
		Are there frequent wrong turns or episodes of getting lost traveling to well-known places (direction sense)?
		Are there frequent problems judging where you are in relationship to objects around you (for example, bumping into things in a dark, familiar room)?
		Is there frequently a problem recognizing objects just by their feel?
		Are left and right often confused?
		Is there frequent trouble learning a new task or skill?
		Parietal Lobe Progression and Severity Totals (add up the total number of checks for this section in each column)
		Total Progression and Severity Scores

Brain Area Questions

Place a check mark in the columns corresponding to the questions that apply to you or the person you are evaluating.

Interpretation

1. Add up your scores in each area and use the key that follows to determine their meaning.
2. Severity Score: defined as the number of abilities or behaviors where there is frequent difficulty. The Severity Score is the number of checkmarks in the left column.
   Severity Score: _____
3. Progression Score: defined as the number of abilities or behaviors that are a lot worse than 10 years ago. The progression score is the number of checkmarks in the right column.
   Progression Score: _____

Interpreting the Severity and Progression Scores

1. If both the severity score and the progression score are 0, then there does not seem to be a problem.
2. If the severity score is 1 or the progression score is 1 and neither of them are 2 or higher, then there may be a very early stage problem or this could be normal aging. If you or others have concern about a problem, then proceed with further testing, such as that suggested in Appendix A. Evaluation for depression should also be done if there is any sad mood or loss of motivation.
3. If either the severity or the progression score is 2 or higher, then the chance of cognitive impairment or dementia is higher. This situation should be further evaluated with the tests described in Appendix A. Evaluation for depression should also be done if there is any sad mood or loss of motivation.

chapter 5

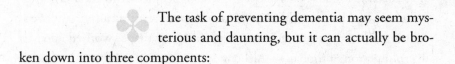

Reduce Your Risk

The task of preventing dementia may seem mysterious and daunting, but it can actually be broken down into three components:

1. Know and reduce the risk factors that are under your control.
2. Have a regular memory screening to detect problems early.
3. Obtain an accurate, early diagnosis and then treatment.

All three of these components go a long way in either preventing or delaying ADRD and its progression, and they ensure that you or your loved ones will lead a full and happy life, even with the presence of the disease.

Knowing what your risks are and taking steps to reduce them is one of the best ways for you to prevent the onset of Alzheimer's disease and related disorders from devastating your life. We are often asked the question "Is Alzheimer's inherited or environmental?" It would be nice if there were an easy answer to the "nature versus nurture" question, but unfortunately there isn't. When people are struck by ADRD, we almost always find that nature and nurture both played a part. Whatever genetic predisposition you have, your genes always operate within the life you lead. Is it healthy or unhealthy, safe or full of risks? Many are born with certain traits and vulnerabilities, but how they conduct their day-to-day lives has a huge impact on how they age and whether they are afflicted by disease. Genes interact with overall health in every way, not just with ADRD. For instance, a person may be prone to high cholesterol and heart disease, but if she eats a healthy diet and exercises, she can maintain her health well into her seventies and eighties. Your genes interact with lifestyle, injuries, medical problems, exposure to toxic substances, diet, and more.

Recognizing your risk early gives you a clear direction on how to conduct your life so that you do *not* cause or encourage the onset of dementia. If you know you are at genetic risk for Alzheimer's disease, you will want to avoid environmental factors that further increase your chances for it. For example, if someone has the apoE4 gene, which increases the risk of AD, he would be well advised to avoid contact sports or activities that increase the risk for head injuries at all costs, because even minor head injuries increase the risk for AD in vulnerable people. Unfortunately, most sports are played during childhood, adolescence, or young adulthood. People this age feel youthful and vital. The last thing they're worried about is "that old person's problem"—Alzheimer's disease. Yet it is precisely at this age when they may start themselves on a downhill slope toward dementia. We believe that children should be screened for the apoE4 gene before being allowed to play contact sports. If they screen positive, they should play golf instead of football, table tennis instead of hockey.

Below you will find a summary of both the genetic and acquired (environmental) risk factors for ADRD. We have evaluated the certainty of each risk factor by examining the quality of the research in the scientific literature, and assigned it to one of five levels according to the criteria of evidence-based medicine (EBM), a process that is gaining popularity in the medical field because it involves asking clear questions of the published scientific literature that ascertains how much results should be trusted. Some of the questions are: What studies have actually been conducted? How good are they? What is the evidence of their validity and clinical usefulness? Have the results of the studies been applied to real patients to ascertain whether specific treatments are effective? Have these patients been tracked over time? It is important to review how these studies are conducted and backed up to evaluate their significance to you.

EBM Level 1: Group Studies—Highest Reliability

Group studies select their subjects from the general population before the researchers know whether or not the subjects have any risk factors at all. Researchers then evaluate for a particular risk factor by studying these randomly selected individuals. This type of study is considered to have the highest level of reliability because selecting from the population as a whole reduces bias and offers a clearer picture of what is true for all people. Subjects are divided into groups according to age, gender, race, occupation, and so on, and they are followed for a period of years to determine the probability within the grouping of developing a particular ADRD disease.

EBM Level 2: Case-Control Studies—Second-Highest Reliability

These studies randomly select from two groups of individuals: those who already have dementia and those who do not. Researchers then test to find out the percentage of people in each group who have a particular risk factor—either environmental or genetic—and come up with what is called the "relative risk" of the average person. Case-control studies can be misleading. The risk factor being measured may not be fairly represented in the "cases" (people who have dementia) and "controls" (people who don't have it). A major example of this problem occurred with studies on the risk of cigarette smoking with regard to AD. More than eight case-control studies declared that smoking cigarettes actually reduced the risk of developing AD. However, when the more reliable "group studies" were conducted, they revealed that cigarette smoking either increased the risk or had no effect at all—it certainly didn't reduce Alzheimer's disease. The reason the case-control studies were so misleading is that many cigarette smokers who have Alzheimer's disease simply die earlier than nonsmokers who have it. Consequently, when researchers randomly selected AD patients for their studies, more AD smokers had died.

EBM Level 3: Case Series Studies—Third-Highest Reliability

These studies select a sample of patients who have dementia and calculate what percentage of them happen to have a particular risk factor for dementia. Researchers use this information to determine the relative risk for the general population. But since there is no control group (that is, people who are normal), researchers cannot tell whether nondemented individuals also have the same relative risk. In the aforementioned case of cigarette smokers, a case series study would have concluded (as the case-control studies did, and rather incorrectly) that smoking decreases one's chances of developing AD when in point of fact it increases it.

EBM Level 4: Animal Studies—Fourth-Highest Reliability

There is a certain bonus in conducting animal studies: every aspect of the environment can be controlled. Unfortunately, though, because they are a different species from us, they don't have identical anatomy. What is true for their bodies is not always true for ours. The meaning of any results obtained from tests on an animal can only be inferred for humans. As we have seen in countless newspaper reports, the result of tests conducted on rats often does not hold true for people. For one thing, rats have virtually no prefrontal cortex, while the human prefrontal cortex takes up 30 percent of the brain. The Food and Drug Administration is well aware of this. That is why, after the animal research has been conducted, the FDA requires three more levels of human studies before it approves of any disease treatment. An example of successful animal research that did not work well in human trials was the vaccine against beta amyloid produced by Elan Pharmaceuticals to treat AD. It worked well in animal research but caused brain inflammation in a number of research subjects, and four of them died.

EBM Level 5: Test Tube or Tissue Research— Lowest Reliability

This kind of research looks at the laboratory effect of a treatment on a particular risk factor for ADRD disease. For example, manufacturers of herbs and vitamins have recently researched the effects of particular vitamins or

Table 5.1. ADRD Risks That Cannot Be Modified: Age, Gender, and Genetics			
ADRD (Dementia) Risk Factor	**Relative Risk***	**Type of Dementia**	**EBM Level†**
Age			
65–74	2.0	All	1
75–84	7.0	All	1
85+	38.0	All	1
Gender			
Male	2.0	VD	2
Female	2.0	AD	2
Ethnicity			
African-American, if family history of AD	1.6	VD	1
Caucasian	1	All	
Hispanic	1.5	AD	
Family history			
AD in a First-Degree Relative	3.5	AD	2
AD in 2 or more First-Degree Relatives	7.5	AD	2
Family History of Down syndrome	2.7	AD	2
Apolipoprotein E4 gene (1/2 copies)	2.5/5	Late onset AD	1
Presenilin 1 gene	aut. dom.**	Early onset AD	1
Presenilin 2 gene	aut. dom.**	Early onset AD	1
Down syndrome	aut. dom.**	Early onset AD	1

*Risk of getting ADRD due to the given risk factor compared to persons without that risk factor. Relative risk means the increased chance someone with the risk factor may develop dementia.

†Evidence-based medicine level, which indicates the quality of the research for each of the listed ADRD factors. 1 is the highest quality; 5 is the poorest quality.

**Autosomal dominant. Children of parents with this gene have a 50 percent chance of inheriting the disease.

herbs on the formation of beta amyloid or neuritic plaques in a test tube or in tissue cultures of animal models of AD. Unfortunately for the consumer, if the manufacturers find that the compound reduces beta amyloid or neuritic plaques, they usually stop the research and start selling it to the consumer. As with animal research, there are many reasons why a beneficial effect in a test tube or in tissue culture will not work in humans.

Age, Gender, and Genetic Risk Factors

Age. This is the biggest risk factor for all types of dementia (ADRD). As many as 10 percent of all people 65 years of age and older have ADRD. As many as 50 percent of all people 85 and older have the disease. In the general population, the risk for developing ADRD approximately doubles every 5 years after the age of 65 (34). After age 50 there is also an increased risk for vascular dementia.

Gender. Whether one sex or the other is more susceptible to developing ADRD is unknown because the research is quite conflicting. That said, after an extensive review of the relevant literature, it seems that after the age of 75, the risk of ADRD appears greater in women than in men (35), even accounting for the fact that women live longer than men.

Ethnic background. Deciphering whether there is more or less risk for ADRD in different ethnicities is complicated by other factors: variations in education, genetics, acculturation, and longevity—all of which are factors in and of themselves. To date, all of these factors require further research to determine whether certain groups are more susceptible. Large reviews on the connection between ethnicity and ADRD have led to the following preliminary conclusions (32):

1. There appears to be an increased risk of ADRD in Hispanic Americans and VD in African Americans.
2. The risk of ADRD with an apolipoprotein E4 is about the same for different ethnicities living in the United States including Ashkenazi Jews, African Americans, Hispanic Americans, and Caucasian Americans.

Genetic risk factors. A family history that includes ADRD often does not predict well for an individual. This is especially true for people who have a first-degree relative (mother, father, brother, or sister) with ADRD; they are about three and a half times more likely to develop symptoms. It appears that people with a family history of Parkinson's disease are even more likely to develop Alzheimer's disease or its related disorders. A recent study revealed that people with first-degree relatives with Parkinson's disease were six times more likely to develop dementia than those in the general population.

Beta amyloid depositions are the primary disease mechanism of AD. At least four genetic causes of AD are known to increase BA42 production:

- Inheriting the E4 version of the apolipoprotein E (apoE) gene on chromosome 19, which causes AD to appear later, usually after age 65 (36)
- Overproduction of amyloid precursor protein (APP) by the beta APP gene on chromosome 21, which occurs in Down syndrome and causes AD to appear early, between age 35 and 65, in people with Down syndrome
- Inheriting the Presenilin 1 gene on chromosome 14 (PS1), which causes AD to appear early, between age 35 and 65 (37)
- Inheriting the Presenilin 2 gene on chromosome 1 (PS2), which causes AD to appear early or later, between age 40 and 85 (37)

A chromosome is a threadlike structure found in the nucleus of a cell. It is one giant molecule of DNA, made up of hundreds and sometimes thousands of genes. We all have a set of 23 pairs of chromosomes—one set from each parent—giving us a total of 46 chromosomes. A gene, a very small part of a chromosome, is coded to make different kinds of proteins, which in turn make up your cells, which in turn make up you. A normal person has just the right amount of chromosomes and the right amount of genes on that chromosome. When the number of chromosomes is wrong, or when there are extra genes on a chromosome, or when the genes are out of sequence, problems occur.

The ApoE Gene

Everyone has two apoE genes, and if one of them—or worse, two of them—are apoE4, that person's likelihood of getting ADRD is quite high. Of course, apoE genes alone are not dangerous; we need them to function. They help in the development, maturation, and repair of cell membranes of neurons, and they help regulate the amount of cholesterol and triglycerides in nerve cell membranes. There are three versions of the apoE gene—E2, E3, and E4—and it is the last one that is the culprit. As with all genes, we inherit one copy from each parent, and any person could have one of the following six possible combinations:

1. E2/E2
2. E2/E3
3. E2/E4
4. E3/E3
5. E3/E4
6. E4/E4

If a person has two E4 genes, it means she received one from each parent. Because the apoE4 gene is known to increase the beta amyloid deposition and plaque formation that is found in people with AD, it increases the chance of developing the most common form—late onset Alzheimer's disease—by 2.5 (for one E4) or fivefold (for two E4s) (38). The apoE4 gene also causes symptoms to appear two to five years earlier than for those who don't have it but have some other cause of AD.

For about 15 percent of the general population, at least one of their two apoE genes is the E4 gene. People who have no apoE4 gene at all have only a 5 to 10 percent chance of developing AD after age 65, whereas people with one apoE4 gene have about a 25 percent chance. That is quite a jump. But the good news that can be inferred here is that not everyone with the gene will develop AD; in fact, 75 percent will not. One other thing to consider is that even if a person has one apoE4 gene and develops dementia, Alzheimer's disease might not be the source. There is a chance that the cause of the dementia could be from something else. If a person has two apoE4 genes, on the other hand, and develops dementia, the odds are very, very good that it is from Alzheimer's disease. In fact, the odds are 99 percent.

The Beta APP Gene, Down Syndrome (DS), and Alzheimer's Disease

People who have Down syndrome have three copies of chromosome 21—that's one copy more than everyone else has. On chromosome 21 is the gene that produces APP that eventually gets broken down into harmless fragments, as well as the BA42 protein, the one that accelerates neuritic plaque formation and causes AD. Rather than having two genes that produce APP, people with DS have three genes that produce it. Consequently, they produce one and a half times as much APP as everyone else does. Their body cannot get rid of the excess, and it makes larger amounts of BA42. By the age of 40, all DS persons exhibit the brain changes that are characteristic of AD.

Down syndrome is one of the most common causes of metal retardation in the U.S., with approximately 350,000 people currently suffering from it. Children born with the condition have some degree of mental retardation along with the characteristic physical features. Virtually all DS persons who live to age 65 will develop AD.

The Presenilin Genes (PS1 and PS2) and Alzheimer's Disease

Two other genes, presenilin 1 and 2 (PS1 and PS2), are genetic causes of ADRD. They have been found in families where a number of members have Alzheimer's disease; PS1 is on chromosome 14, while PS2 is on chromosome 1. Both of these gene mutations greatly accelerate beta amyloid production. The PS1 gene causes symptoms to appear when people are between 35 and 65. The PS2 gene is more rare and causes symptoms to appear between age 40 and 85.

Environmental Risks

Many of the major acquired or environmental risk factors for ADRD can be modified.

Alcohol and Drug Abuse

(EBM level 2—increases vascular dementia and possibly AD risk)

Alcohol use is a double-edged sword, as it can increase or decrease risk for stroke, heart disease, VD, and possibly AD (see Chapter 3, page 49) (39). Five percent of all strokes in the United States are alcohol-related. Four or more drinks a day increase risks for stroke, heart disease, and vascular dementia, while one drink every few days reduces these risks (presumably by increasing HDL cholesterol, which clears other types of cholesterol that cause hardening of the arteries). Interestingly, studies show that people who do not drink alcohol at all have a higher risk of death from stroke or heart disease.

Clearly, drug abuse damages the brain. There are more than a hundred brain-imaging studies that demonstrate that drug abuse—including that of cocaine, methamphetamines, marijuana, heroin and other opiates—diminishes brain function and damages neurons. One of the first things Dr. Amen learned from doing his brain imaging on a wide variety of psychiatric patients was that drug abuse damages the function seen on SPECT scans. He has made several posters that hang in over 10,000 schools, prisons, and drug abuse treatment centers nationwide on the effects of drugs on brain function. Recently, it was found that cocaine inhibits a part of cells that is involved in energy production; this same finding has been linked to Parkinson's disease.

Reducing Risk and Effects

Alcohol abuse is a major risk factor for stroke and therefore VD, and drugs clearly damage brain function. Preventing abuse of these substances is critical to reducing the risk of dementia. Alcoholism and drug abuse tend to run in families. People with a family history of substance abuse tend to have either too much brain activity or too little ability to calm it on their own. When there is too much activity they tend to use substances that calm brain function, such as alcohol, marijuana, or opiates. When there is too little activity in their brains they tend to self-medicate by using substances that stimulate brain function, such as cocaine or methamphetamines. These findings are clearly seen on SPECT scans. The overactive areas tend to be in the limbic or emotional brain (often associated with depression), basal ganglia (often associated with anxiety), and anterior cingulate gyrus (often associated with worry and obsessions). The underactive areas of the brain are most often seen in the prefrontal cortex and temporal lobes, associated with illness such as attention deficit disorder and learning disabilities. Because their brains are excessively active or inactive, "hot" or "cold," people seek ways to calm or stimulate the activity. Drinking alcohol is the most socially acceptable way to settle down the "hot" spots. Using excessive caffeine, nicotine, and cocaine are ways people stimulate brain activity. There are better, more efficient, and less toxic ways to balance the brain.

A variety of behavioral methods have a balancing effect on brain function. Yoga, meditation, tai chi, hypnosis, biofeedback, and soothing music tend to calm the brain, while physical exercise and more intense music tend to stimulate it.

Diets high in refined sugars—such as those found in candy, pastries, and soda pop—are likely to increase brain excitation and increase the uncomfortable symptoms that at-risk people experience. A more balanced diet, like that recommended in Barry Sears's book *The Zone*, is a good approach to eating that balances brain function. Seeking the aid of a nutritionist or dietitian can be helpful.

If behavioral and dietary methods do not work, then there are medications such as Neurontin, Gabatril, Topamax, Tegretol, Depakote, Trileptal, and Inderal, which can reduce the amount of brain excitation or increase calming or inhibition. For example, 10 mg of Inderal (propranolol) is used by many concert performers to reduce stage fright. There are also medications that help stimulate the brain—psychostimulants such as Adderall or Concerta and stimulating antidepressants such as Wellbutrin and Effexor.

In general, it is best to avoid tranquilizers and sedatives in the class of drugs called benzodiazepines (i.e., Valium, Ativan, Xanax, Serax, Restoril, and Halcion) to calm the brain because tolerance develops after daily use for about one month, and one requires increasing doses to get the same effect. As the dose of a benzodiazepine is increased, it is more likely to cause confusion or memory loss. SPECT studies show marked overall decreased activity with these medications, which can be calming but also leave you cognitively impaired.

It is important to realize that alcohol and drug abusers will always want to overconsume alcohol or other substances because of the genetically programmed imbalance between too much or too little brain excitation. Rather than try to "tough it out," which rarely works, it is better to seek an alternative method of treatment that balances brain function.

In addition to the behavioral methods already mentioned, there are many effective behavioral treatment programs to help one quit alcohol or drugs if abuse develops. Some of these include Twelve Step programs such as Alcoholics Anonymous, individual alcohol and drug abuse counselors, and substance abuse treatment programs offered by many hospitals.

If you cannot stop on your own, there is a medication that makes you sick if you drink alcohol (Antabuse) and one that significantly decreases the high from alcohol (Naltrexone). There are also medications that help for other forms of substance abuse. Also, the medications previously mentioned can be used to balance the brain and reduce the need to use. Finally, alcohol or drug abuse is often associated with other neurological conditions, such as attention deficit disorder (ADD), depression, obsessive-compulsive disorder, and anxiety disorder. Having a psychiatrist or other drug treatment specialist evaluate for these conditions and treat identified problems will reduce the need to use harmful substances.

Cancer and Cancer Treatment

(EBM level 3—increases ADRD risk)

In addition to cancers that invade the brain and can cause dementia, the treatments for cancer that get into the brain can also cause dementia. However, there are few studies on this issue. One of these studies examined the effect of chemotherapy in 100 women with breast cancer. Dr. van Dam found that women who received chemotherapy plus tamoxifen were 4 to 8 times more likely to develop cognitive impairment than women with early stage breast cancer who had not received chemotherapy (40). A review of children who are long-term survivors of cancer, particularly medulloblastoma and acute lymphocytic leukemia, showed that the two most common long-term effects of radiation therapy and chemotherapy are cognitive and hormonal impairment. Surprisingly, they found that the cognitive impairment is progressive and not static. Anything you do to decrease the risk of cancer will also help your brain stay healthy.

Reducing Risk and Effects

Reduce your risk of cancer by avoiding excessive exposure to the sun, stopping smoking, exercising, and eating right. According to guidelines from the American Cancer Society, smoking cessation, diet, and exercise are important ways to decrease cancer risk. They recommend that you

- Eat a variety of healthful foods, with an emphasis on plant sources.
- Eat five or more servings of a variety of vegetables and fruits each day.
- Include vegetables and fruits at every meal and for snacks.
- Limit french fries, snack chips, and other fried vegetable products.
- Choose whole grains in preference to processed (refined) grains and sugars.
- Limit consumption of refined carbohydrates, including pastries, sweetened cereals, soft drinks, and sugars.
- Limit consumption of red meats, especially those that are processed and high in fat.
- Choose fish, poultry, or beans as an alternative to beef, pork, and lamb.
- When you eat meat, select lean cuts and smaller portions.
- Prepare meat by baking, broiling, or poaching rather than frying or charbroiling.
- Choose foods that help maintain a healthy weight.
- When you eat away from home, choose food low in fat, calories, and sugar and avoid large portions.
- Eat smaller portions of high-calorie foods. Be aware that "low-fat" or

"fat-free" does not mean "low-calorie" and that low-fat cakes, cookies, and similar foods are often high in calories.
- Substitute vegetables, fruits, and other low-calorie foods for calorie-dense foods such as french fries, cheeseburgers, pizza, ice cream, dough-nuts, and other sweets.

The American Cancer Society also recommends that people adopt a physically active lifestyle. Here are some tips they recommend to be more active:

- Use stairs rather than an elevator.
- Walk or bike to your destination, if possible.
- Park away from stores and shopping areas.
- Exercise at lunch.
- Go dancing.
- Wear a pedometer every day and watch your daily steps increase.
- Use a stationary bicycle while watching TV.
- Plan your exercise routine to gradually increase the days per week and minutes per session.

In preventing cancer, it is important to maintain a healthful weight throughout life. Being overweight or obese is associated with an increased risk of developing several types of cancer such as breast (among post-menopausal women), colon, uterus, esophagus, gallbladder, pancreas, and kidney.

Alcohol is an established cause of cancers of the mouth, pharynx (throat), larynx (voice box), esophagus, liver, and breast. Alcohol may also increase the risk of colon cancer. People who drink alcohol should limit their intake to no more than two drinks per day for men and one drink a day for women.

Cardiovascular Disease

Cardiovascular disease is a major risk factor; it includes the following types.

Atherosclerosis

(EBM level 1—increases VD and AD risk)

Atherosclerosis is the buildup of fatty cholesterol deposits called plaques on the inside walls of arteries. As plaques build up in an artery, the artery gradually narrows and can become clogged. As an artery becomes more and more narrowed, less blood can flow through. The artery may also become less elastic (called "hardening of the arteries"). Atherosclerosis is the main cause of a group of diseases called cardiovascular diseases— diseases of the heart and blood vessels. In persons with the apolipoprotein E4 gene, there is an increased risk of coronary artery disease, high cholesterol, and AD (41). Surprisingly, having coronary artery disease per se does not increase your chance of developing dementia (42). However, if coronary artery disease is not well controlled, it will lead to either low or high blood pressure, heart attack, and stroke, all of which increase risk for both AD and VD. The most common risks for developing atherosclerosis are high blood cholesterol levels, especially high LDL ("bad cholesterol") or low HDL ("good cholesterol"), age, being male (women are affected more after menopause), high blood pressure, diabetes, smoking, trouble managing stress, obesity, physical inactivity, and having close relatives who had heart disease or a stroke at a relatively young age.

Reducing Risk and Effects

The most effective way to prevent atherosclerosis is to prevent the diseases that produce it. Exercise and diet are all important factors that you have some control over. You can also investigate your family history. If it includes heart disease, stroke, diabetes, high cholesterol, peripheral vascular disease, or alcohol abuse, then you should consult your physician and ask her to screen for these conditions at the appropriate age of risk for the condition, or after age 40 in general. An annual screening after age 50 is extremely wise. Regular cardiovascular exercise for 30 minutes or more 4 to 5 times a week goes a long way to improve lipid metabolism and to reduce lipid deposits in blood vessel walls. The main focus of your diet should be to not overdo it on saturated fats that are high in the bad cholesterols and that contribute to the fatty deposits in the blood vessels that cause atherosclerosis. Foods high in saturated fats include butter, cheese, cookies, doughnuts, pastries, ice cream, fatty meat, and so on.

Once atherosclerosis has developed, the most effective method of prevention to keep your condition from worsening is to have your physician *identify and treat all the underlying causes of it*. Statins—such as Lipitor, Mevacor, and Zocor—have been recently identified as effective treatments to reduce atherosclerosis from elevated LDL or reduce total cholesterol levels (see Chapter 6, page 152, for specific recommendations).

Atrial Fibrillation

(EBM level 1—increases VD and AD risk)

Atrial fibrillation is a fluttering of the heart (arrhythmia) that reduces the amount of blood it can pump. The fluttering of the heart also allows blood clots to form, which are then pumped into the bloodstream. Atrial fibrillation is a well-known risk factor for stroke and vascular dementia. When atrial fibrillation causes blood clots to form, they flow through narrower and narrower vessels and sometimes clog the vessel completely. If the clot does not dissolve quickly, using the blood's natural anticlotting mechanisms, the tissue downstream dies. This is one of the mechanisms of a stroke. The fluttering heart during atrial fibrillation also reduces blood flow to the brain and starves its deepest areas, which accumulate small strokes over a period of years. These deep white matter areas control leg movement. If they are damaged, slowing of movement, incoordination, unsteadiness, or loss of balance will develop. With more severe atrial fibrillation, strokes accumulate in larger areas of the deep white matter and result in mental slowing or even Parkinson's-like symptoms.

Reducing Risk and Effects

If you have a family history of any kind of irregular heart rhythm, including a heart that beats too fast (tachycardia) or too slow (bradycardia), then your physician should check you regularly after the age of 40 to 50 with an electrocardiogram or whatever is the most appropriate screening test at the time.

If you do not have atrial fibrillation or other irregular heart rhythms, preventing them from occurring involves keeping the heart healthy. Just like all other cells, cardiac cells function best when they receive adequate input, which means adequate blood flow and periodic stimulation, both of which are accomplished by regular exercise.

Anyone who has heart palpitations, fluttering, or symptoms of unexplained lightheadedness or dizziness should be evaluated for an irregular heart rhythm. If you have atrial fibrillation, then you can minimize its harmful effects with proper medical treatment. The pacemakers that are called "demand pacemakers" can be very helpful. They sense when your heart rhythm is irregular and attempt to electrically correct the rhythm. Coumadin, a powerful blood thinner, is routinely used in atrial fibrillation to prevent blood clots and strokes, although some patients with mild forms of atrial fibrillation are not treated.

People with atrial fibrillation should have a brain MRI, SPECT, or PET scan on a regular basis to determine if small strokes are accumulating or if AD is developing. If so, then the atrial fibrillation should be more aggressively treated to prevent or delay the onset of VD and AD.

Carotid Bruit

(EBM level 1—increases VD risk)

Carotid bruit is a condition caused by narrowing of the carotid artery, which increases VD risk. The carotid arteries in your neck supply blood to most of your brain. The term *bruit* is French for "noise" and refers to the whooshing sound the carotid artery makes when it becomes narrowed by disease. When a carotid artery becomes too narrow, the brain may not receive enough blood, and a stroke can occur. The major causes of carotid bruits are atherosclerosis, hypertension, and diabetes.

Reducing Risk and Effects

See the section on atherosclerosis, page 89, for prevention strategies. Carotid bruits can be treated medically or surgically. Coumadin is the primary medical treatment when the carotid bruit indicates a severely narrowed artery that is likely to cause stroke. For lesser degrees of narrowing, baby aspirin, Ticlid, Plavix, Aggrenox, and Persantine are all used in various combinations. At present, it appears that Aggrenox is the most effective treatment to reduce stroke risk and VD (Aggrenox is a combination of baby aspirin and long-acting Persantine). Carotid endarterectomy is a surgery that can bypass the blockage of a severely narrowed carotid artery.

Congestive Heart Failure

(EBM level 1—increases VD risk)

Congestive heart failure (CHF) is the last stage of many forms of heart disease. When the heart muscle becomes too weak to pump blood efficiently, blood backs up in the body, and swelling can occur as blood flow become congested. Heart diseases such as coronary artery disease, atrial fibrillation, and diseases affecting the heart valves all can ultimately produce CHF if not treated effectively. With CHF the heart is less efficient in pumping blood to the brain.

Reducing Risk and Effects

The most effective way to reduce the risk of VD due to CHF is to prevent it by treating its underlying causes effectively. Just as first detecting and treating a person when she is moderately demented is much less effective than treating her early on, the same is true for CHF.

Coronary Artery Disease

(EBM level 1—increases VD and AD risk)

Coronary artery disease (CAD) is a major cause of heart disease, which is one of the two leading causes of death among adults in the United States and other developed countries; CAD is also the primary cause of heart attacks. Atherosclerosis is the primary cause of CAD (see the earlier section on atherosclerosis). Because CAD is a form of atherosclerosis, it increases AD risk, presumably through increasing BA42 to accelerate neuritic plaque formation.

Reducing Risk and Effects

Proper exercise, diet, annual screening, and some medications can help. See the section on atherosclerosis, page 89, for further recommendations.

High Cholesterol (Hyperlipidemia)

(EBM level 1—increases VD risk and possibly AD risk)

High total or LDL (low-density lipoprotein) cholesterol is a well-known risk factor for stroke and heart disease, both of which are risk factors themselves for vascular dementia. However, high total or LDL cholesterol may also increase risk of AD. As part of the U.S.A. Women's Health Initiative research, a group of 1,037 women under 80 years old with coronary artery disease who did not have a hysterectomy were studied for four years. This study found that elevated levels of either total or LDL cholesterol almost doubled the risk for memory loss, cognitive impairment, or dementia. Lowering total and LDL cholesterol into the normal range eliminated this increase in risk. Although most normal ranges for total cholesterol include values below 200, levels below 180 have been associated with less atherosclerosis and a better outcome. Lowering cholesterol below normal values can cause aggression, so cholesterol should be kept within the normal range.

Reducing LDL cholesterol may reduce neuritic plaque formation in AD by reducing the number of LDL receptors in nerve cell membranes. Fewer LDL receptors reduce the amount of BA42 beta amyloid cleared from neurons, which reduces neuritic plaque formation and delays AD progression. This is particularly important in people with an apoE4 gene.

Reducing Risk and Effects

People with a family history of high cholesterol should consider getting an apoE genotype blood test. Because of the accelerated neuritic plaque production associated with the interaction between apoE4, BA42 beta amyloid, and the LDL receptor, if you have an apoE4 gene, then it is even more important to keep your LDL cholesterol levels from elevating. Cardiovascular exercise and a healthy diet improve lipid metabolism to help keep your cholesterol levels normal. Statins such as Lipitor and Zocor are the most effective treatments to reduce total and LDL cholesterol. The liver synthesizes most of the cholesterol around bedtime, so these medications should be taken then. Statins also reduce AD risk in people under 80 by as much as 75 percent (see the section on statins in Chapter 6, page 152, for specific recommendations).

Hypertension (High blood pressure)

(EBM level 1—increases VD risk)

Hypertension is a well-established major risk factor for stroke, heart disease, and VD. In hypertension, chronically elevated pressure on blood vessel walls causes the muscle cells to enlarge and stiffen, thus narrowing the blood vessels, much as in atherosclerosis.

Reducing Risk and Effects

Hypertension can run in families. If you have a family history of hypertension, stroke, or heart disease, get your blood pressure checked on a regular basis. Early intervention is essential to ward off the untoward long-term effects. The most effective way to prevent hypertension, or to minimize it if you already have it, is to do 30 minutes of cardiovascular exercise at least every three days, and preferably daily.

A number of studies have shown that biofeedback can reduce mild hypertension. Biofeedback is based on the very simple concept that if you receive feedback on a physiological process in the body—such as breathing, hand temperature, sweat gland activity, heart rate, or blood pressure—then over time you can learn to exert control over those processes.

The proper control of blood pressure is essential to reducing the risk of further strokes and VD. People with prior stroke who maintain their systolic blood pressure (the top number in blood pressure readings) between 135 and 150 mm Hg reduce their risk for future strokes and VD. Lowering systolic blood pressure below 135 may be beneficial for some patients but not for others. For some people lowering blood pressure too much reduces blood flow to the brain and increases stroke risk. Those individuals who probably should not lower their blood pressure below 135 usually have more severe, long-standing hypertension or have symptoms of lightheadedness or dizziness when standing, getting out of bed, or changing positions too quickly.

Cerebral Vascular Disease (Brain Blood Vessel Disease)

Cerebral vascular disease includes both stroke and TIAs (see below).

Stroke

(EBM level 1—increases the risk of VD)

The risk of developing vascular dementia in a person who has a stroke is 6 to 10 times greater than that of the general population (43). Even a stroke smaller than a pencil-head eraser (called lacunar infarct, *lacune* means "little lake") increases the risk for vascular dementia 4 to 12 times. In people who have brain changes consistent with AD, whether they have symptoms or not, a lacunar infarct increases the risk of them becoming demented by 20 times. Clearly, stroke is a major risk factor for dementia.

Reducing Risk and Effects

A stroke is a single, damaging attack, but the risk factors that lead to a stroke, such as high blood pressure, smoking, heart disease, and diabetes, develop over a long time. You can reduce your stroke risk by taking the following simple steps:

- Keep blood pressure under control. Check your blood pressure often, and if it is high, follow your doctor's advice on how to lower it. Treating high blood pressure reduces the risk for both stroke and heart disease.
- Stop smoking. Cigarette smoking is linked to increased risk for stroke and heart disease. The risk of stroke for people who have quit smoking for two to five years is lower than for people who still smoke.
- Exercise regularly. Exercise makes the heart stronger and improves circulation. It also helps control weight. Being overweight increases the chance of high blood pressure, atherosclerosis, heart disease, and adult-onset (type 2) diabetes. Physical activities like walking, bicycling, swimming, and tennis lower the risk of both stroke and heart disease. Talk with your doctor before starting a vigorous exercise program.

- Eat a healthy, balanced diet and control diabetes. If untreated, diabetes can damage the blood vessels throughout the body and lead to atherosclerosis.

The warning signs for stroke are: sudden numbness or weakness in the face, arm, or leg, especially on one side of the body; sudden confusion, trouble speaking or understanding; sudden trouble seeing in one or both eyes; sudden trouble walking, dizziness, loss of balance or coordination; sudden severe headache with no known cause. If you suspect that either you or someone you know is having a stroke, call 911 immediately, even if the symptoms seem to have gone away. Sometimes the warning signs last for only a few minutes and then they disappear, but that does not mean the problem is resolved. You could have had a transient stroke, called a transient ischemic attack (TIA—see the next section), and although it doesn't last long, it is a symptom of a greater medical problem. Don't ignore a TIA—see your doctor right away.

Transient Ischemic Attack (TIA)

(EBM level 1—increases risk of VD)

Transient ischemic attacks, better known as TIAs, are strokes that reverse themselves, usually within an hour but always within 24 hours. This reversal does not mean a TIA is harmless. The disappearance of a symptom only means that enough circuit damage has been repaired to resume normal function. It does not mean that all the damage has been reversed. The appearance of a TIA is just the tip of the iceberg; it is symptomatic of the final stage of damage to a brain circuit that tells us something is wrong. As we have mentioned, with subcortical VD, brain imaging can show thousands of accumulated small strokes that did not produce the sudden onset of any symptoms; TIAs are therefore a major warning sign of greatly increased risk for stroke and vascular dementia. In fact, if a patient has more than two TIAs over a period of months, physicians will treat him or her with Coumadin (the most potent anticoagulant of all), because the risk of stroke is so high.

Reducing Risk and Effects

A TIA indicates significant underlying disease of either the heart or blood vessels from the heart to the brain. Atherosclerosis is usually the condition affecting blood vessels that causes TIAs, as well as heart disease, carotid bruits, and others. The most effective way to prevent TIAs before they occur is to reduce the chance of heart disease and atherosclerosis. The most effective prevention, once a TIA occurs, is to have your physician *identify and treat all the underlying causes of your TIA*. This involves evaluation for heart disease and atherosclerosis, and treatment of the identified conditions. Baby aspirin (81 to 175 mg daily) is commonly used to reduce the risk of stroke and vascular dementia.

Depression

(EBM level 1—increased risk for ADRD)

A prior history of medically treated depression can be associated with a threefold increase in the risk of ADRD. In an impressive study, Doctors Kristine Yaffe and Terri Blackwell at the University of California, San Francisco, studied the association between depression and cognitive decline (44). As part of an ongoing prospective study, they evaluated 5,781 elderly women. They studied them at baseline and four years later, using tests of depression, memory, and concentration. At baseline, 211 (3.6 percent) of the women had six or more depressive symptoms. Only 16 (7.6 percent) of these women were receiving treatment, which meant that 93.4 percent of the depressed women in the studied group were not being treated. Increasing symptoms of depression was associated with worse performance at baseline and follow-up on all tests. Women with three to five symptoms of depression had 1.6 greater odds for cognitive deterioration, and women with six or more symptoms of depression had 2.3 greater odds for problems—more than double the risk. The researchers concluded that depression in older women is associated with both poor cognitive function and subsequent cognitive decline.

It is critical to note that most psychiatric diseases in general are, in effect, brain diseases. Schizophrenia, for example, has been shown to affect the frontal and temporal lobes, and depression has shown decreased activity in the frontal lobes. These illnesses are also exacerbated by chronic stress; increases in stress hormones have been shown to kill cells in the hippocampus.

Reducing Risk and Effects

Early treatment is essential to stave off the ravages of psychiatric illnesses. Our work with SPECT teaches us that with appropriate treatment, the brain becomes more balanced and works in a much more efficient way. Treatment can be with medication, psychotherapy, supplements, or a combination of all three. Medication and supplements work by altering certain neurotransmitters in the brain; for example, antidepressants work by enhancing serotonin, norepinephrine, or dopamine. Psychotherapy has also been shown recently to affect neurotransmitter systems and enhance the activity seen on SPECT and PET scans.

Diabetes

(EBM level 1—increases risk for VD and impairs function in AD)

Diabetes damages almost every organ, including the brain, by making blood vessels hard and brittle. This increases the likelihood of stroke, heart disease, and hypertension, all of which increase VD risk.

In diabetes there is a failure to keep blood sugar (glucose) at appropriate levels, which impairs memory and other cognitive functions in people with dementia. If a person already has dementia, controlling blood glucose is still beneficial, in that it improves memory and other cognitive functions. Sometimes the treatment of diabetes lowers blood glucose too much (hypoglycemia), which can also impair memory and other cognitive functions.

Reducing Risk and Effects

People with a family history of diabetes should have a fasting blood glucose test once a year after the age of 40. In addition, if symptoms of increased urination, increased thirst, or increased appetite develop, then fasting blood glucose should be checked for diabetes. One of the most effective preventions of diabetes is exercise, which improves the ability of insulin to regulate blood glucose. Although there are many reasons that daily exercise is better than exercise every three days, the available data suggest that exercising at least every three days helps protect against diabetes and a number of other illnesses. Diets high in refined sugars increase the risk of diabetes. A balanced diet such as that recommended in *The Zone,* by Barry Sears, is a good approach to eating that helps stabilize blood sugar. Consulting with a nutritionist or dietitian is also a good idea.

People with well-controlled diabetes can live a full and normal life. In addition to the proper diet and exercise, there are many effective medications to treat diabetes and keep elevated blood glucose from damaging your blood vessels and organs. The long-term level of glucose control can also be monitored and adjusted with a blood test called HbA1c.

Education and Occupation

Education and occupation also play a part in one's risk of getting ADRD.

Less Than Eighth-Grade Education

(EBM level 1—increases risk for ADRD)

Having less than an eighth-grade education is a risk factor for developing ADRD after age 75 (35). A number of studies that attempted to identify risk factors for dementia have noted an inverse relationship between education and dementia: the more education, the less dementia. This is a controversial risk factor, because educational background and achievement can introduce a number of other factors that generally affect health and opportunity. Despite the controversy, there is significant evidence to support the idea of education (and increased mental activity) producing a functional reserve in the brain, which is a process that can provide protection against developing dementia. As we have mentioned, long-term potentiation (LTP) is the neuronal correlate of learning and memory; LTP reduces the sensitivity of hippocampal neurons to overstimulation from the neurotransmitter glutamate and seems to protect neurons from the effects of acute lack of oxygen.

The principle of "Use it or lose it" is very much at play in the brain. The more it is challenged and stimulated (without overdoing it, which leads to the harmful effects of stress), the more ability it will have as we age. No one that we are aware of has studied whether or not learning disabilities and other conditions, such as attention deficit disorder, that often lead to school failure are associated with ADRD. Our strong suspicion is that there is a connection. Any condition that negatively impacts brain function can put the brain at risk for other problems later on. We believe in aggressive treatment of children and teenagers with school problems so that they will stay in school and perhaps learn to love learning and be the lifelong learners they need to be to help protect their brains.

Reducing Risk and Effects

Keeping your mind active by reading, doing crossword puzzles, traveling, taking classes, and otherwise acquiring knowledge outside of your typical or usual experience helps to reduce the risk of dementia.

And don't ignore learning problems in children and teenagers, hoping they will disappear on their own. They must be addressed early and vigorously. Adults also should pay attention to any learning difficulties they may experience. Over 15 years ago it was assumed that only children had learning disabilities and attention deficit disorder, and adults were somehow immune. In fact, many adults suffer from these problems as well, and no matter how old they are, they can benefit dramatically from treatment. If you have trouble with reading, writing, listening, paying attention, or being organized, seek an evaluation from a competent professional. It could change your life.

Occupation: Unskilled Jobs with No New Learning

(EBM level 1—increases risk for ADRD)

There is also an increased risk for workers who have an unskilled job with no new learning required. In many ways the brain is like a muscle. It needs to be used and stimulated in order to maintain the tone that is essential for health and fitness. People in rote, routine, or boring jobs often go for long hours without cerebral challenge or stimulation and leave for home cognitively worse than when they came to work.

Reducing Risk and Effects

If you find yourself in this situation, try to upgrade the skill level of your job. If changing jobs is not possible or practical, then after work, compensate for your brain's "down time" by pursuing hobbies or outside interests that require new learning. With all the adult-education classes available, myriad possibilities exist: you can take on a language, try a new game that makes you think, take a class in computers, join a literature group, or learn about a subject that has always interested you.

Lack of Exercise

(EBM level 1—increases the risk of dementia)

Exercise has profound and broad-based effects on your health. The Honolulu Aging Asian-American Study examined risk factors of diabetes, high cholesterol, high blood pressure, and heart disease among 215 men in their fifties, and then followed them for 36 years to determine who became demented. The men with the higher number of risk factors were much more likely to develop vascular dementia (45). Since all of these risk factors can be minimized by regular exercise, the risk of vascular dementia can be lowered by regular cardiovascular exercise. The Honolulu Aging Study also found that men who exercise less than twice a week in their forties are more likely to become cognitively impaired or demented after age 70. A study done at Case-Western Reserve University looked at how much TV people watch each day, which correlates with their exercise level. People who watched two or more hours of TV a day (couch potatoes) were twice as likely to develop AD. In contrast, people over 40 years old who exercise at least 30 minutes per session, two or more times a week, can expect the following benefits:

- After the age of 70, their memory and other cognitive abilities are less likely to be impaired.
- There is an increase of DNA repair in their cells.
- There is an increase of blood flow to the brain, as well as more efficient oxygen and glucose metabolism.

- The brain is protected against molecules that overexcite it, including free radicals, too much glucose, and too much glutamate.
- There is improved brain metabolism of cholesterol and other lipids.
- The ability of insulin to regulate glucose remains efficient.
- The response of neurons (in the hippocampus at least) to physical stress is better.
- The tone in blood vessels is improved because appropriate levels of nitric oxide are maintained.

Animal research suggests even more profound benefits of exercise. Rats running on an exercise wheel showed the following benefits after a single session:

- Their brain-derived neurotrophic factor (BDNF) levels were raised for three days, which enhanced their short-term memory (via enhancing LTP).
- New neurons were generated in the hippocampus and frontal cortex and this new generation persisted for four weeks.
- Synaptic connections between neurons were formed and strengthened, which improved brain function in general.

The data on exercise is impressive and incontrovertible. Our distant ancestors exercised as part of daily life when they hunted and gathered food, fled their enemies, and tracked down a mate. In the modern world where we sit in a cubicle in front of a computer screen all day, then come home at night and slump in a recliner to watch TV, we have to make an effort to do what our ancestors did as a matter of course. Our bodies did not evolve to be motionless and inert; they evolved so that the muscles, heart, and cardiovascular system need to be activated.

Reducing Risk and Effects

The greatest obstacle most people have in committing to regular exercise is making it a habit. People don't think twice about brushing their teeth, showering, dressing, or adjusting the rearview mirror when they climb into the car, because these activities are all habits that they've trained their brains to perform automatically. From your brain's perspective, a habit is a series of actions it executes when you tell it to do so fairly automatically and without effort. But it requires many repetitions before your brain learns to automatically perform a function. Think of how many times it took before you learned to ride your bike without training wheels. The real challenge of exercise is to train your brain to make it into a habit.

The best chance of making exercise a habit, therefore, is to schedule a specific time and place to exercise each day or at least on specific days each week. Consider using the same shoes and clothing and doing the workout in the same place, but have a variety of exercises to choose from so you can vary the routine. The idea is to exercise consistently according to schedule for the first few months. After several months, you will find that you no longer think about whether you want to get out there and work out or not. When you reach that point, it has become a habit, one that will keep you healthy and save you more money than any other single thing you ever do for your health. It's well worth the effort.

Head Trauma

(EBM level 2—increases risk for AD tenfold if one has the apoE4 gene [32])

However, without an apoE4 gene, a head injury does not increase the risk of AD. This means that of the 2 million people in the USA per year who have a head injury, one-quarter of those who lost consciousness (up to 500,000 people) are 10 times more likely to develop AD.

Head injury itself can cause cognitive impairment or dementia, particularly when there is loss of consciousness or repeated head injuries (see Chapter 3). The effects of head injury can worsen over time as scar tissue forms within the areas of the brain that were hurt.

Studies using SPECT scans have shown that there is healing after a brain injury. If a SPECT study shows problems right after the injury, it does not necessarily predict how bad things may be down the line. The brain has many natural healing mechanisms. If, however, a SPECT study shows damage nine to twelve months after an injury, then the problems are likely to be permanent, without intense intervention. When symptoms worsen after the first year, there is almost certainly something else going on that needs to be diagnosed and treated.

Head Trauma and High-Contact Sports

Head trauma and the risk of AD is a particularly serious and neglected problem among professional athletes in high-contact sports such as football, hockey, soccer, rugby, and boxing. Few studies have examined whether such athletes are more likely to develop AD. About one-quarter of these athletes have an apoE4 gene, and almost all of them have had at least one head injury with unconsciousness. National Football League quarterbacks such as Steve Young and Troy Aiken, who have suffered multiple concussions, are at particularly high risk for AD if they have the apoE4 gene. It is estimated that chronic traumatic brain injury occurs in approximately 20 percent of professional boxers. It is often termed dementia pugilistica, or DP. The risk for DP increases with duration of career, age of retirement, total number of bouts, poor performance, increased sparring, and the presence of the apoE4 gene; DP shares many characteristics with Alzheimer's disease (i.e., neurofibrillary triangles, diffuse amyloid plaques, acetylcholine deficiency, and/or abnormal tau proteins).

Reducing Risk and Effects

Given the extraordinary increase in risk of AD when a head injury is added to the presence of the apoE4 gene, it would be wise to know your apoE genotype before you engage in high-risk activities. If you discover that you have a gene that predisposes you to Alzheimer's disease, you will almost certainly be motivated to find an alternative sport to engage in—one where you won't get struck in the head. The knowledge will also stimulate you to use what you now know to delay the onset of and progression of AD through prevention, early detection, diagnosis, and treatment. Your actions will have a direct effect on keeping you out of a nursing home and reducing the burden on your loved ones. You can also plan more realistically for the future of your children by knowing their genetic predisposition because you can guide them away from activities likely to cause brain injuries that could devastate their lives years after you are gone.

If you decide to get an apoE genotype blood test, then it should be done under the strictest confidence so that insurance companies or others cannot obtain this information and potentially use it against you. It would be best to pay for the test on your own and keep it in your personal records but not allow it to be included in your medical records.

Those who should consider getting an apoE genotype blood test include:

- Those who are considering playing contact sports where there is a high risk of injury to the head
- All professional athletes who engage in high-contact sports (boxing, football, soccer, hockey, etc.)
- Those with a brother, sister, father, or mother with AD
- People who have sustained a head injury with loss of consciousness or who have had multiple head injuries

For those who have already sustained a head injury and wish to reduce their risk of permanent consequences, as well as for those who engage in activities with a high chance of incurring a head injury, it may be useful to consider the daily use of antioxidants, plus an anti-inflammatory medication, because free-radical generation and brain inflammation contribute to the damage caused by trauma to the brain.

A well-designed longitudinal study in the Netherlands found that people who eat food high in the antioxidants—vitamins C and E (basically fruits and vegetables)—reduce their AD risk by 20 percent (5). Antioxidants can block the kind of brain damage that is caused by the free-radical production occurring after head trauma. Free radicals damage DNA and turn on a self-destruct program called apoptosis—programmed cell death. Animals subjected to brain trauma showed considerably less brain damage if they were fed a high-antioxidant diet consisting of blueberries, garlic, and spinach *before* the trauma. And a diet high in antioxidants *after* head injury could help and certainly would not hurt.

Taking vitamins or herbal compounds to obtain higher doses of antioxidants may be beneficial. For example, ginkgo biloba, a potent antioxidant, has been studied in rats given moderate head injury. Ginkgo given to the rats up to 17 hours after the head injury did not reduce brain swelling, but it did markedly reduce the number of free radicals produced by damage to nerve cell membranes (46). These free radicals significantly contribute to the brain damage caused by head injury. Alpha lipoic acid is a powerful antioxidant that increases the potency of other antioxidants to minimize brain damage by free radicals. Alpha lipoic acid has not been studied in head trauma, but at doses of 600 mg per day it successfully treats painful diabetic neuropathy, the damage of which is partly caused by free radicals.

As almost all professional athletes in high-contact sports know, non-steroidal anti-inflammatory drugs (NSAIDs) reduce joint and tissue swelling if they are taken before or immediately after a game. Head injury causes brain inflammation and swelling too, so NSAIDs can reduce it if they are taken before or shortly after the trauma. Because head injury can accelerate BA42 beta amyloid formation in people with an apoE4 gene, ibuprofen, sulindac, and indomethacin may be more effective than other NSAIDs, since they are the only ones known to reduce beta amyloid formation (in animal models) (47). (See Chapter 6 for specific NSAID recommendations.)

The cognitive impairment caused by a head injury may be more damaging if left untreated, because when a particular type of functioning is diminished, one is unlikely to force oneself to engage in activities that utilize the part of the brain involved in that function. In other words, that part of one's brain will be dormant. Neurons or their connections that are not periodically activated wither away from disuse, a process known as use-dependent plasticity, or "Use it or lose it."

Dr. Arnold Scheibel and his colleagues at the University of California, Los Angeles, reported a fascinating example of use-dependent plasticity (48). They examined the brains of 20 neurologically normal men and women with varying levels of schooling who died in their forties or fifties. In particular, they looked at the area of the brain that helps us understand language (Wernicke's area). Those who had had more education or who engaged in more mentally stimulating activity had neurons that looked bushier, with larger branches than those with less education or less mental stimulation during their lives. The effects observed on the neurons of these individuals were not genetic; they were primarily the result of using the mind through education and "mental exercise." In other words, when a brain area is used more, its neurons get bigger, stronger, healthier, and more resistant to damage from a variety of causes.

This finding has important implications for those who have had a head injury. A head-injured person may avoid activities that depend on the function of the damaged brain areas, such as reading, writing, or learning. However, using the damaged brain area causes its neurons to shrink and wither away even further, thus magnifying the original damage. Therefore, the best way to regain the abilities that have been damaged by head injury is to start using them again. This is a lot easier if the person receives the proper medical treatment and rehabilitation therapy. We have treated many brain-injured patients who recovered much more once they received the proper treatment.

Homocysteine

(EBM level 1—increases the risk of VD and AD)

Homocysteine is an amino acid regulated by folic acid in red blood cells. If elevated, homocysteine increases risks for coronary artery disease, stroke, and vascular dementia. Furthermore, analysis of the Framingham study showed that AD risk doubles for homocysteine levels greater than 14. The risk is largely eliminated for homocysteine levels of 10 or below (49).

High homocysteine levels in the blood increase LDL cholesterol, which narrows the coronary blood vessels of the heart to produce what is called coronary artery disease. Coronary artery disease leads to heart attacks, stroke, and vascular dementia if not effectively controlled by diet, exercise, and medication. A study of persons who required the opening up of their coronary arteries in a procedure called coronary angioplasty showed that homocysteine levels higher than 11 could be treated with folic acid (1 mg), vitamin B_{12} (400 mcg), and pyridoxine (10 mg) to reduce the levels to about 7. This homocysteine reduction helped prevent renarrowing of the coronary arteries after the angioplasty surgery and halved the chance that these blood vessels would close up again and require another angioplasty surgery (50). In addition, high homocysteine levels can make blood clot more easily than it should, increasing the risk of blood vessel blockages and stroke or heart attack.

Homocysteine is normally changed into other amino acids for use by the body. If your homocysteine level is too high, you may not have enough B vitamins to help this process. Most people with a high homocysteine level don't get enough folate (also called folic acid), vitamin B_6 (pyridoxine), or vitamin B_{12} in their diet. Replacing these vitamins helps return the homocysteine level to normal. Other possible causes of a high homocysteine level include low levels of thyroid hormone, kidney disease, psoriasis, some medicines, or inherited deficiencies in the enzymes used to process homocysteine in the body.

Reducing Risk and Effects

Like many diseases, high blood levels of homocysteine can run in families. If you have a family history of stroke, VD, or AD, then it is a good idea to have your blood homocysteine levels checked every few years after the age of 40 or 50, which is when vascular disease begins to affect the brain.

Homocysteine is measured using a simple blood test. It can be measured at any time of day. It is not necessary to prepare in any special way for the blood test (such as fasting). Most hospital labs can measure homocysteine, or a blood sample can be sent out to a special lab. A healthy homocysteine level is less than 10 micromoles (μmol) per L (liter). A level higher than 10 μmol per L is considered high and should be reduced.

While no studies have proved that lowering homocysteine levels ultimately helps reduce strokes, heart attacks, and other cardiovascular events, it is a good idea to lower a high homocysteine level because it is a risk for heart disease.

Eating more fruits and vegetables (especially leafy green vegetables) can help lower your homocysteine level by increasing the amount of folate you get in your diet. Good sources of folate include many breakfast cereals, lentils, chickpeas, asparagus, spinach, and most beans. Folate is sometimes called folic acid.

If adjusting your diet is not enough to lower your homocysteine, you will also need to take specific vitamins. You may need to take a fairly large amount of folate (about 1 mg per day). Additional vitamin B_6 and vitamin B_{12} also help the body process homocysteine. The usual recommended vitamin and folate doses for lowering homocysteine levels are as follows:

- A daily multivitamin containing 400 mcg (micrograms) of folate
- An additional 800 mcg of folate per day for 8 weeks

If taking these vitamins doesn't lower your homocysteine level, your doctor may have you try a higher dose. Or you may need to have some tests to see if you have a health condition that causes high homocysteine levels.

Hormones

Hormones also play a part in one's risk for ADRD.

Estrogen Deficiency Induced by Menopause

(EBM level 2—may increase risk of AD)

Six of ten studies showed that women who took estrogen had a lower risk for AD. The best of these studies were EBM level 1. In the Baltimore Longitudinal Study of Aging (51), 472 women who were going through menopause or had completed it were followed for up to 16 years. Women who never used estrogen during the study were twice as likely to develop AD.

This study and others showing a beneficial effect of estrogen have been recently contradicted by reports from the Women's Health Initiative, which found that women who used Premarin (an estrogen made from horse ovaries) were twice as likely to develop AD as those who did not use estrogen. However, the Women's Health Initiative study did not examine the risk of AD using forms of estrogen made by the human ovary, such as estradiol. Evidence suggesting that these more natural forms of estrogen for women may still reduce AD risk and provide other benefits comes from the largest study ever done on the severest form of estrogen deficiency— hysterectomy with removal of the ovaries (52). This study of 100,000 women who participated in the 1986 National Mortality Followback Survey found that women with a hysterectomy were twice as likely to develop dementia due to ADRD. What one can conclude from this complex maze of seemingly contradictory research findings is that women should avoid

Premarin and other forms of estrogen that are not made by the human ovary. However, severe reductions in female estrogen hormones are equally harmful and should be treated. There is a large body of basic scientific research demonstrating sound reasons why estrogen, in the right amount, protects the brain, the blood vessels, and the bones. Human forms of estrogen, taken in the smallest amounts needed to keep blood estradiol levels from falling too low in women after menopause, are reasonably safe and have not, to date, been demonstrated by the Women's Health Initiative or any other study to be harmful.

Reducing Risk and Effects

If there is a family history of AD, then it is worth having a blood estradiol test after menopause to determine if you have estrogen deficiency. You can then evaluate with your doctor whether low-dose estradiol or other natural estrogens would be worth taking. The situation is more complex in women with a family history of AD and breast or uterine cancer, because estrogen use increases the risk of these two cancers. Whether low-dose estradiol significantly increases the risk of heart disease or stroke in women without symptoms is more controversial. The relative benefits of taking low-dose estradiol after menopause (reduced risk of AD and osteoporosis) may be greater than the relative risks (increased risk of endometrial cancer, breast cancer, and maybe stroke and heart disease), but the decision regarding treatment depends on your personal history and the risk factors for each of these diseases.

Although not all studies agree, estrogen use after menopause appears to significantly reduce AD risk. Estrogen use in estrogen-deficient women can also improve verbal fluency and possibly verbal short-term memory. Evista is a form of estrogen that is safer to take in women with increased risk of breast or uterine cancer.

Hysterectomy Without Hormone Replacement

(EBM level 1—doubles the risk of ADRD)

Dr. Shankle and his colleagues examined the most severe form of estrogen deficiency in women—hysterectomy with removal of the ovaries followed by no estrogen supplementation—to see if dementia risk was increased. Not giving estrogen after hysterectomy was the standard of care in the United States during the 1960s, 1970s, and 1980s. His group analyzed the data on over 100,000 women who were part of the National Mortality Followback Survey. This is the largest population-based study ever done, and it clearly showed a twofold increase in dementia among women with hysterectomy compared to those without. This study did not distinguish the different causes of dementia, so we don't know whether severe estrogen deficiency increases just AD risk or other ADRD risks as well.

Reducing Risk and Effects

If your ovaries have been removed by hysterectomy or other means, then you should consider taking low-dose estradiol under your physician's guidance. You would no longer be at risk for uterine cancer, because hysterectomy removes it. While the risk for breast cancer, heart disease, and stroke may be increased with low-dose estradiol or other natural estrogens, the risk of dementia may be higher, especially if you have a family history of dementia or the apoE4 gene. This is a complex decision that we hope will become clearer as further data become available on the effects of low-dose estradiol and the natural estrogens. Evista is a safer alternative treatment for those women with combined risk for dementia and breast cancer.

Testosterone Deficiency in Men

(EBM level 2—increases risk of dementia)

Testosterone deficiency itself produces impairment in visual memory and visual spatial abilities. Reduced testosterone levels also lower estradiol levels, which lead to impaired working and short-term memory. Testosterone levels normally start to decline after age 50. By age 80, testosterone levels are 20 to 50 percent of their younger adult values.

Low testosterone levels may increase AD risk. A case-control study involving 83 AD patients and 103 normal volunteers of similar age showed significantly reduced total testosterone levels in AD males. However, until a well-designed group study is done, it is not certain whether testosterone deficiency is a risk factor for AD.

Reducing Risk and Effects

Men who have or have had prostate cancer treatment or men age 50 and older may develop cognitive impairment due to testosterone deficiency, which can be checked by a blood test. Symptoms of difficulty with vision not due to eye problems, difficulty remembering locations or faces or other objects of interest, breast enlargement, or a change in the distribution of body hair should alert one to check for testosterone deficiency. An AD patient of Dr. Shankle's was treated with Lupron injections for prostate cancer and had a testosterone level of zero. Treatment with enough testosterone to normalize his testosterone level improved his visual spatial abilities.

Parkinson's Disease

(EBM level 2—increases risk for ADRD)

Parkinson's disease is caused by the loss of dopamine-producing cells. There is a significant connection between PD and AD.

Reducing Risk and Effects

There is no known cure for PD, but with early detection there are medications that help with the symptoms. It has also been suggested that coenzyme Q10, a powerful antioxidant, along with high doses of vitamin C may be helpful in delaying the need for stronger and stronger medications. Vitamin B$_6$ increases the production of dopamine and may be helpful early in the disease process. The natural hormone melatonin, which regulates sleep, has been found to reduce tremors and protect against free radical damage on dopamine neurons. Fish oils and flaxseeds contain omega-3 fatty acids, which have nerve-nourishing effects that can boost dopamine.

Hypnosis may also be helpful to reduce tremor in PD. When Dr. Amen was a resident at the Walter Reed Army Medical Center in Washington, D.C., he wrote a scientific article on a patient with Parkinson's disease who benefited from hypnosis. It has been known for some time that the tremor associated with PD is markedly lessened during sleep. Dr. Amen noticed that when he put this patient in a hypnotic trance his tremor went away. It happened over and over, and was videotaped and presented at the weekly grand rounds lecture. Several other patients also benefited from hypnosis. The theory of why hypnosis was helpful was that there might be a connection between hypnosis and sleep. Another theory was that stress increases the symptoms associated with PD and hypnosis induces a relaxed state. If learned early, deep relaxation techniques may be helpful in reducing the ill effects of PD.

Seizures and Seizure Medication

(EBM level 3—increased ADRD risk)

A seizure may be convulsive or nonconvulsive. It may last only a few seconds or a few minutes. It may produce automatic behavior, or uncontrollable shaking movements. It may be just a blank stare. It may be no more than a strange feeling in which things look, sound, or taste different from what they really are.

No matter how different they look on the outside, all seizures are the same on the inside. They are all produced in the same way—by a sudden, brief malfunction in the delicate electrical system of the brain. Differences in what the seizures look like depend on what part of the brain is affected and whether the misfiring is limited to just one area or involves the whole brain. These dramatic events show up as sharp spikes in brain wave patterns recorded by the electroencephalograph (EEG).

About 125,000 Americans develop epilepsy every year. Thousands more experience isolated seizures that may or may not happen again in the future. Recurring seizures are defined as epilepsy. Treatment of epilepsy has improved dramatically in recent years. Seizures can often be controlled, and chances of long-term remission are improving all the time.

Seizures and certain antiseizure medications can have a negative effect on brain function and be associated with ADRD. During seizures there is dramatic increased activity seen on SPECT and PET studies. In the in-between period, there is significant decreased activity. Antiseizure medications work by increasing inhibition in the brain. If this is done too enthusiastically, as with the older antiseizure medications like Dilantin and phenobarbital, it can cause overall decreased activity and damage the healthy cells around the seizure-promoting ones.

Reducing Risk and Effects

Obviously, seizure disorders need to be vigorously treated. Once a person is seizure-free for two years, however, many neurologists, start to taper the antiseizure medications to see how much is needed. And newer antiseizure medications, such as Trileptal, are less likely to cause too much overall inhibition of brain function. If you are taking antiseizure medication and notice memory problems, that is a symptom that the temporal lobes may be calmed too much.

However, the most common cause of seizures in someone with epilepsy is not taking seizure medication as prescribed. For some people whose seizures cannot be controlled with medication, there is surgery to take out the damaged tissue. Brain SPECT is used in many centers to help pinpoint the seizure area. Most surgery takes place in people whose seizures begin in one fairly small part of the brain that can be removed without affecting speech or memory or some other important brain function. Operations to prevent seizures from spreading from one side of the brain to the other or to remove large areas of one side of the brain are also performed.

The diet that has been successful in preventing seizures is called the ketogenic diet, akin to the Atkins low-carbohydrate diet. It is used most often for children who, for one reason or another, cannot take the standard medications.

Sometimes it is possible to identify a certain action or event that will always produce seizures in sensitive people. Seizure "triggers" include flickering lights, breathing very quickly and deeply, drinking an excessive amount of fluid, and even, in very rare cases, reading or listening to a certain piece of music. Sleep deprivation (like staying up all night studying) may produce seizures; so may excessive use of alcohol or withdrawal from certain drugs. Avoiding seizure triggers may require no more than a slight readjustment of activities. For example, making sure there's plenty of light in the room when playing video games or watching TV and covering one eye when approaching the set to change channels have been recommended for people with special sensitivity to TV flicker. Polarizing sunglasses may help when the flickering of reflected sunlight is a problem. Lack of sleep, extreme fatigue, excessive dieting, exposure to extreme heat in showers or tubs or from excessive exertion on very hot days, or even emotional stress may trigger seizures in susceptible people. The best way to prevent that from happening is to follow basic rules of good health—sufficient sleep, staying active, eating a healthy, balanced diet, and, if you take seizure-preventing medicine, not letting yourself miss doses or run out of medication.

Sleep Apnea

(EBM level 3—increased risk of ADRD)

Obstructive sleep apnea—a condition associated with loud snoring, stopping breathing entirely for brief periods many times during the night, and chronic tiredness—can cause cognitive impairment. The only brain SPECT study of obstructive sleep apnea examined 14 moderate to severely affected patients, who stopped breathing more than 30 times per hour. Their brain SPECT scans showed significantly reduced activity only in the left parietal lobe (53). Reduced left parietal lobe activity can impair comprehension, making it difficult to understand conversations or read books.

Figure 5.1. Sleep Apnea SPECT

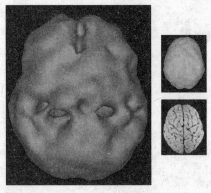

Top view
Decreased parietal lobe activity

Table 5.2. Environmental, Acquired, and Modifiable Risks for ADRD

Dementia (ADRD) Risk Factor	Relative Risk*	Type of Dementia Affected			EBM Level†
		AD	VD	Multiple Types	
Alcohol and Drug Abuse					
Alcohol abuse (> 4 glasses/day)	4.4	X			2
Alcohol abuse (> 4 glasses/day)	2.45		X		2
Beer drinkers v. non–beer drinkers	2.0			X	
Cancer and cancer treatment					
Standard-dose chemotherapy for breast cancer	3.5			For cognitive impairment	2
High-dose chemotherapy for breast cancer	8.2			For cognitive impairment	2
Cardiovascular disease					
Atherosclerosis (hardening of the arteries)	2.0	X	X		1
Atrial fibrillation	1.5		X		1
Carotid bruit (narrowing of blood vessel in the neck)	2.0	X	X		1
Congestive heart failure with low blood pressure	1.3		X		1
Coronary artery disease	2.5		X		1
Heart attack (myocardial infarction) AND female	2.9	X	X		2
Hyperlipidemia (high total or LDL cholesterol)	2.1	X	X		1
Hypertension: systolic blood pressure > 180 mm Hg	2.3		X		1
Relative low blood pressure: systolic blood pressure lowered below 135 mm Hg if previously hypertensive	1.8–2.5		X		2
Cerebral vascular disease (brain blood vessel disease)					
Stroke	10		X		1
Small strokes (lacunar infarcts)	4–12		X		1
Small strokes *plus* AD	20	X			3
TIA: transient ischemic attack	4.8		X	X	1
Depression					3
Depression, 3–5 symptoms	1.6			X	
Depression, 6 or more symptoms	2.3			X	

Dementia (ADRD) Risk Factor	Relative Risk*	Type of Dementia Affected				EBM Level†
		AD	VD	Multiple Types		
Education/occupation						
Less than eighth-grade education	2.0			X		1
Unskilled occupation (little learning involved)	2.0			X		2
Exercise						
Exercise less than twice a week	2.0	X				3
Head injury						
Head injury with unconsciousness or multiple head injuries	2.0			X		2
Head injury with unconsciousness AND 1 or 2 apolipoprotein E4 genes	10.0	X				2
Homocysteine level						
High blood levels	2.0	X	X			2
Hormones						
Estrogen use after menopause	2.0	X				2
Hysterectomy with ovary removal	2.0	X	?			1
Testosterone	1.3	X				3
Parkinson's disease						
Parkinson's disease	3.0			X		2
Seizures and seizure medication	1.5					2
Sleep apnea	not known					3
Smoking						
Smoking	2.3	X	X			1

*Risk of getting ADRD due to the given risk factor compared with persons without that risk factor. Relative risk means the increased chance that someone with the risk factor may develop dementia.

†Evidence-based medicine level, which indicates the quality of the research for each of the listed ADRD risk factors. 1 is the highest quality; 5 is the poorest quality.

Treatment of the sleep apnea with nasal continuous positive airway pressure (CPAP, a machine that pushes air at a high pressure through the nasal passageways) completely reversed the impaired brain activity in these patients. Dr. Amen recently evaluated a man with severe sleep apnea who had memory complaints. The brain SPECT scan showed almost no activity in his parietal lobes. Treating his sleep apnea with CPAP significantly improved his memory.

Reducing Risk and Effects

Sleep apnea should be evaluated and treated as early as possible. The warning signs of sleep apnea include loud snoring; witnessed pauses in breathing; awakening while gasping for breath; falling asleep at inappropriate times during the day; irritability; trouble with attention, concentration, comprehension, or memory; headaches upon awakening; frequent nighttime sweating and urination; or even occasional episodes of bedwetting. If you have any of these, get a sleep evaluation and do not ignore the treatment suggestions.

Smoking

(EBM level 1—smoking cigarettes increases VD Risk)

Cigarette smoking accounts for 12 percent of all the strokes in the United States and is therefore a major risk factor for vascular dementia (31). Tobacco constricts small blood vessels in the cortex and can cause small cortical hemorrhages. By constricting small cortical blood vessels, tobacco also reduces blood flow to the white matter and basal ganglia so that these areas become progressively damaged over a period of years.

Smoking does not reduce AD risk! While a large number of case-control studies found that cigarette smoking actually reduced the risk for AD (through the effect of nicotine), this was later found to be wrong when more statistically valid group studies were performed. Ironically, nicotine itself turns out to help improve memory loss and other cognitive impairments in people with mild dementia. Nicotine may also have a disease-delaying effect by blocking programmed cell death, although this has only been shown in animal studies so far.

Reducing Risk and Effects

Obviously, stop smoking. We know for many this is easier said than done. Over the years Dr. Amen has helped many, many people stop smoking. No one program works for everyone. Hypnosis is effective for some, the use of nicotine patches or gum works for others, the medication Wellbutrin (bupropion), a dopamine-enhancing antidepressant, is helpful for others, and some respond to group therapy. In our experience it is usually a combination of treatments that are needed. As we have shown, however, smoking is a risk factor for many of the illnesses related to ADRD, and stopping is essential, even more so if you have the apoE4 gene.

As we have shown, there are many risk factors associated with ADRD. There are, however, common themes to cutting the risk for these very serious disorders. The risk-reducing measures are consistent with an overall healthy lifestyle, such as not taking risks for brain injury, stopping smoking, avoiding too much alcohol, eating a healthy diet, and exercising on a regular basis. In the next chapter we will go into more detail on specific prevention strategies.

chapter 6

Steps to Prevention

After a review of the medical research into preventive strategies, we both take vitamin E, vitamin C, and low-dose ibuprofen every day. Despite being very busy physicians, we also exercise daily for 30 minutes or more and try to eat right, including eating fish, fruit, and vegetables. Dr. Shankle, who has strong genetic ADRD risk factors—such as diabetes, stroke, heart disease, and high cholesterol—inherited from both sides of his family, reduces these risks further by taking ginkgo biloba and alpha lipoic acid twice daily.

We take the preventive actions because we believe there is enough research to support using each of these agents to reduce our ADRD risks. Furthermore, these preventive strategies are safe if a physician annually monitors them for potential side effects. The key to health and longevity is using safe prevention strategies as early as possible. If we wait until all of the answers to preventing ADRD are firmly established before we apply safe strategies, we will already be affected.

> *Your physician should monitor your prevention strategies on a yearly basis.*

Preventive therapies can postpone the onset of ADRD by six years and probably more. We will provide you with an objective rating of the scientific research behind each preventive agent discussed in this chapter, so that you know how likely it will be to actually reduce your specific ADRD risks. In the United States, manufacturers of some products make statements that mislead consumers into thinking that the product has been proven to prevent a specific disease. It is hard for the average consumer to know what really helps. For example, we see some patients who take 20 different supplements and have no way of knowing whether they really help them, harm them, or simply make manufacturers rich. Because there is a wide range of "proof of benefit" of these supplements and strategies, we have indicated the level of evidence for their effectiveness.

You do not need to do all of the recommended prevention strategies. Evaluate each of them for your own personal situation and risk factors. Unless there is a reason not to, we recommend that everyone engage in regular mental and physical exercise, take vitamins C and E, fish oil, and low-dose aspirin or a nonsteroidal anti-inflammatory drug.

Acetyl-L-Carnitine (ALC)

Recommended	Probably, if well tolerated
Level of evidence	Good
ADRD risk reduced	Heart disease, stroke
Amount risk reduced	Not yet defined
Suggested dose	1,000–2,000 mg per day
Suggested monitoring	None

About 95 percent of cellular energy production occurs in the mitochondria. Many diseases of aging are increasingly being referred to as mitochondrial disorders. The biologically active amino acid involved in the transport of fatty acids into the cell's mitochondria for the purpose of producing energy, ALC is sold in Europe to treat heart and neurological disease. It can increase muscle mass and convert body fat into energy. It has been shown to protect brain cells against aging-related degeneration and to improve mood, memory, and cognition. Many people use ALC to maintain immune competence and reduce the formation of the aging pigment lipofuscin. The most important effect of ALC, however, is to maintain the function of the cell's energy powerhouse, the mitochondria.

In analyzing a multisite study (24 sites) with 334 patients with Alzheimer's disease, Dr. J. O. Brooks at Stanford University found that ALC significantly slowed the progression of Alzheimer's disease in younger subjects (54). Also, several Italian studies, including more than 130 patients, showed that ALC improved memory, verbal fluency, and attention.

In addition, ALC has been found helpful for a number of illnesses that are risk factors for ADRD, such as stroke, the cognitive impairment from chronic alcoholism, and depression.

Alcohol

Recommended	Yes, if can control alcohol intake
Level of evidence	Excellent
ADRD risk reduced	Heart disease, stroke, dementia
Amount risk reduced	70 percent
Suggested dose	1–2 glasses of wine or spirits, no more than 3 to 4 times a week
Suggested monitoring	Annual checkup after age 50 for heart disease, stroke, hypertension, high cholesterol, gastrointestinal and liver diseases

Alcohol as a preventive strategy needs to be cautiously recommended and is certainly not for everyone, particularly those who cannot control the amount they drink once they start. Many alcohol-related medical problems occur when alcohol is overused, including alcoholic dementia, diabetes, hypertension, high cholesterol, heart disease, stroke, liver disease, cancer, and others. As a prevention strategy, alcohol should only be used by people who can control their drinking to one or two glasses of alcohol, no more than three to four times a week.

Drinking these small amounts of alcohol helps reduce stroke, heart disease, and dementia, probably by preventing atherosclerosis and thinning the blood. Small amounts of alcohol

- Keep platelets in the blood from clotting inside blood vessels and causing a stroke (which is why too much alcohol can cause a hemorrhage)
- Increase HDL (good cholesterol) levels by about 12 percent (about the same as can be achieved with daily exercise or eating fruits and vegetables); the increased HDL reduces the number of LDL (bad cholesterol) molecules to help keep the arteries from getting hard and brittle

Heart disease, stroke, and alcohol. More than 60 prospective studies support the finding that the use of as little as one drink a week of wine, beer, or hard liquor reduces the risk of heart disease and reduces the risk of stroke by about 20 percent (55). In contrast, drinking more than three glasses of alcohol a day is not good for you. It counteracts the beneficial effects of smaller amounts of alcohol and increases the risks of alcoholic heart disease, brain hemorrhage, hypertension, irregular heart rhythms such as atrial fibrillation, throat cancer, pancreatitis, sudden death, and possibly Alzheimer's disease.

For those people who can control their drinking, drinking wine or spirits once a month, once a week, perhaps more than once a week but definitely not daily *can significantly reduce the chance of becoming demented by up to 70 percent, as well as reduce risks of heart disease and stroke* (56). However, if you cannot control your drinking, then don't use this potential benefit of alcohol as an excuse to drink. There are many other ways to reduce your ADRD risks for dementia.

Alpha Lipoic Acid

Recommended	Probably
Level of evidence	Fair
ADRD risk reduced	Diabetes, stroke, solid cancers, programmed cell death
Amount risk reduced	Not yet defined
Suggested dose	300 mg twice a day
Suggested monitoring	None

Alpha lipoic acid (ALA) is powerful antioxidant that increases the potency of many other antioxidants, including vitamins C, E, and, most important, glutathione. Glutathione, the most powerful antioxidant in cells, acts to regulate the cell's ability to absorb free radicals and prevent damage, which has been demonstrated in studies in blood, skeletal muscle, and liver cells. Alpha lipoic acid is a small molecule that readily enters the brain to protect it from free-radical damage.

The research on ALA in ADRD is minimal but promising. In rat cortex, ALA protects neurons from free-radical damage induced by beta amyloid and hydrogen peroxide (a free radical) (57). There is one small human study of nine AD patients given ALA for one year, which showed delayed AD progression; it is currently under investigation by the multi-center Alzheimer's Disease Cooperative Study Unit.

In other types of disorders that are risk factors for ADRD, ranging from cancer to AIDS, ALA has shown significant benefits with varying levels of scientific support. For solid tumor cancers, ALA has been shown to improve survival rate and reduce treatment-related toxicity. In one study ALA reduced the size of strokes by as much as 50 percent (58). In another study ALA improved removal of lead from animal brains poisoned by lead. At doses of 600–1,200 mg per day, ALA significantly reduces leg pain in diabetics for at least two years and improves heart function in diabetics for at least four months. It reduces programmed cell death and reduces AIDS virus activation.

Aspirin

Recommended	Yes, if well tolerated
Level of evidence	Excellent
ADRD risk reduced	AD, heart attack, stroke, peripheral vascular disease
Amount risk reduced	30 percent to 55 percent
Suggested dose	Less than 175 mg per day
Suggested monitoring	Annual physical to check for blood in stool and kidney function and bruising
Notes	Do not take in addition to another NSAID, such as ibuprofen; take one or the other

Aspirin is one of a larger class of medications called nonsteroidal anti-inflammatory drugs (NSAIDs). Aspirin has three primary effects:

- In low doses (175 mg a day or less) when taken for two or more years, aspirin reduces the beta amyloid found in diffuse plaques, which accumulate in all brains with age, but much more so in AD. Some well-designed studies have found aspirin to be as effective as other NSAIDs in reducing AD risk by approximately 55 percent; other studies have shown no effect of aspirin; and other studies show about a 30 percent AD risk reduction (59).
- It keeps platelets from sticking together to prevent clotting inside blood vessels, which protects against insufficient blood flow to all parts of your body, as well as against heart attack and stroke.
- It reduces pain and fever caused by inflammatory cells.

Why do the various well-designed studies show different results in reducing AD risk with aspirin? The answer may in a chemical called nitric oxide. Aspirin, as well as several other NSAIDs, does not stimulate the release of nitric oxide, while other NSAIDs, such as ibuprofen, do. Recently, it was discovered that nitric oxide stimulates the brain's immune cells to remove beta amyloid from the neuritic plaques of AD. This discovery may explain why NSAIDs that do not trigger nitric oxide release are ineffective in treating AD once symptoms have developed. In other words, once AD symptoms have developed, many neuritic plaques have accumulated, and the beta amyloid molecules inside them are resistant to aspirin and most other NSAIDs, except ibuprofen and the other ones discussed later in the NSAID section. This discovery may also explain the disagreement between the various studies on aspirin and AD: the risk reduction in these studies would have depended on the amounts of neuritic plaques in the brains of each "normal aging" population sampled.

In conclusion, low-dose aspirin, for example 81 mg a day (baby aspirin), reduces risk of stroke, heart attack, and peripheral vascular disease and is very likely to reduce risk of AD in people without symptoms. The degree to which AD risk is reduced if you do not have symptoms probably depends on the number of neuritic plaques that have already accumulated when you begin taking aspirin.

If you take aspirin, and wish to also take an NSAID such as ibuprofen, then it is probably wise to alternate them. In other words, take half an adult aspirin with food one day, alternating with a low dose of an NSAID the next day. If memory problems are already present, they may not be helped by an NSAID, although their progression may be delayed. In that case, get an accurate diagnosis and treatment.

Cat's Claw (sold under the name Cogno-Blend)

Recommended	No
Level of evidence	Poor; test tube studies
ADRD risk reduced	Possibly AD
Amount risk reduced	Not yet defined
Suggested dose	Not yet defined

Cat's claw (*Uncaria tomentosa*) is a plant found in South America, the inner bark of which contains compounds that in test tubes block the formation of the toxic form of beta amyloid. It is currently being marketed as Cogno-Blend as a possible preventive agent for AD. At present, there is no evidence that it actually reduces AD risk in humans. The company says that they are conducting trials in humans, but none have been reported to date.

At present, we do not recommend cat's claw or Cogno-Blend to prevent or treat AD until there is at least some reputable human clinical trial evidence that it truly reduces AD risk or delays AD onset.

Choline/Lecithin

Recommended	No
Level of evidence	Poor; animal studies only
ADRD risk reduced	None
Amount risk reduced	None
Suggested Dose	N/A

Choline and compounds derived from choline, such as lecithin, serve a number of vital biological functions. They are involved in cell wall membranes, cell signaling, nerve impulse transmission, and fat metabolism. It has been hypothesized that choline might be helpful to improve memory. Increased dietary intake of choline very early in life can diminish the severity of memory deficits in aging rats. Choline supplementation of the mothers of unborn rats, as well as rat pups during the first month of life, leads to improved performance in spatial memory tests months after choline supplementation has been discontinued. The significance of these findings to humans is not yet known.

More research is needed to determine the role of choline in the developing brain and whether choline intake is useful in the prevention of memory loss or dementia in humans. As we have discussed, AD has been associated with a deficit of the neurotransmitter acetylcholine in the brain. One possible cause is a decrease in the enzyme that converts choline into acetylcholine in the brain. Large doses of lecithin (phosphatidylcholine) have been used to treat patients with dementia associated with Alzheimer's disease in hope of raising the amount of acetylcholine available in the brain. However, a systematic review of the research trials did not find lecithin to be more beneficial than placebo in the treatment of patients with dementia or cognitive impairment.

Coenzyme Q10 (CoQ10)

Recommended	Yes
Level of evidence	Good
ADRD risk reduced	Parkinson's disease, possibly Lewy body disease
Amount risk reduced	44 percent
Suggested dose	1,200 mg/day if symptoms; 100–400 mg/day if no symptoms

CoQ10 is an enzyme that lives inside the mitochondria of your cells and helps convert oxygen into usable cellular energy, called adenosine triphosphate (ATP). Organs that use a lot of oxygen are your heart, muscles, kidneys, pancreas, and brain. If the mitochondria of these oxygen-demanding organs do not properly convert oxygen into energy, they can be damaged. Recently, it was discovered that mutations of the alpha-synuclein gene on chromosome 4 produce Parkinson's disease, a movement disorder that affects about 1 percent of all people over 50 years old. Alpha-synuclein helps regulate the activity of CoQ10 in the mitochondria. In people with PD, CoQ10 activity is reduced in the brain area that causes the problems with movement. Furthermore, reduced CoQ10 blood levels are found in people with Lewy body dementia, a more widespread form of PD.

In animal models of PD, giving CoQ10 actually prevents loss of the affected neurons. A recent multicenter trial of 80 persons with early-stage untreated PD examined the effect of placebo versus 300, 600, or 1,200 mg CoQ10 per day for 18 months (60). CoQ10 delayed the progression of PD symptoms by 44 percent; 1,200 mg per day slowed the decline in movement better than lower doses. CoQ10 may be a safe and effective way to delay the severely debilitating movement disorder of PD.

Since Lewy body disease has the same pathology as PD, except that it has spread to the cortex, CoQ10 may very well delay onset and progression of Lewy body disease (there are no human trials yet on the effects of CoQ10 in Lewy body disease). In AD and VD, blood levels of CoQ10 are not reduced; CoQ10 therefore does not appear to reduce risk for AD or VD.

People with PD or Lewy body disease or a positive family history of these disorders should consider taking CoQ10. If symptoms are already present, then 1,200 mg per day is an effective dose. In people without symptoms, lower doses are probably effective, but the exact dose is not established. A safe dose for people without symptoms is 100–400 mg per day.

Dehydroepiandrosterone Sulfate (DHEA)

Recommended	No
Level of evidence	Poor
ADRD risk reduced	None, and may increase obesity and prostate and breast cancer
Amount risk reduced	N/A
Suggested dose	N/A

DHEA is a steroid involved in testosterone and estrogen production; levels vary widely across individuals and decrease with aging. To date, low DHEA levels are not linked to any specific health disorder. At present, there is no clear reason to support using DHEA to prevent any disease, and there are several good reasons not to take DHEA. The side effects of DHEA are acne and increased facial and body hair, increased lipid (fat) production, and increased risk of hormone-dependent cancers of the prostate and breast. In aging men, DHEA levels do not affect whether they have narrowing of the arteries (atherosclerosis). Among nonsmoking women age 40, lean women have, among other things, lower DHEA levels.

Diet That Is Calorie Restricted and High in Omega-3 Fatty Acids and Antioxidants

Recommended	Yes, unless there is a good reason not to
Level of evidence	Excellent
ADRD risk reduced	Dementia, diabetes, high cholesterol, coronary artery disease, high blood pressure, stroke, obesity, and possibly certain forms of cancer
Amount risk reduced	30–50 percent
Suggested dose	Fruits, vegetables, fish, fish oil supplements if needed
Suggested monitoring	Annual monitoring for coronary artery disease, fasting lipid panel, fasting glucose, high blood pressure, weight

All of your body's cells must be periodically replaced. To do so requires proper nutrition. We all have experienced the effect food can have on our waistlines as well as our mood. If you have doughnuts for breakfast, 30 minutes later you feel blah. A few hours after a huge pasta meal you feel tired and listless. The wrong diet makes you feel bad, and the right diet can help you feel good. Diet is an important prevention strategy. Giving the body essential nutrients effectively helps you rebuild your cells and stay healthy.

Calorie Restriction

Substantial research in animals and now in humans indicates that a calorie-restricted diet is helpful in many ways. It controls weight; decreases risk for heart disease, cancer, and stroke from obesity (a major risk factor for all of these illnesses); and triggers certain mechanisms in the body to increase the production of nerve growth factors, which are helpful to the brain.

Dr. Jose A. Luchsinger and his colleagues at Columbia University in New York examined the association between calories, fat, the apolipoprotein E4 gene, and developing AD (61). They followed 980 elderly normal aging individuals for four years and measured their daily calorie and fat intake. Compared with people with a low calorie or fat intake, those with the highest calorie or fat intake were 2.3 times more likely to develop AD, only if they also had the apolipoprotein E4 gene. Otherwise, the amount of fat and calories made no difference in the risk for developing AD.

In the well-designed Rotterdam study, researchers found that diets high in saturated fat and cholesterol increased dementia risk, while fish consumption decreased dementia risk. They evaluated the food intake of 5,386 normal aging persons and followed them for 2.1 years (5). Those with high intake of total fat, saturated fat, or cholesterol were, respectively, 2.4, 1.9, and 1.7 times more likely than those with lower intake to develop dementia. Vascular dementia was more related to total or saturated fat. Eating fish reduced dementia risk, especially that due to Alzheimer's disease. Clearly, less is more when it comes to diet. In addition to calorie restriction, eating diets high in fish and antioxidants is likely to be very helpful.

Fish, Fish Oil, and Omega-3 Fatty Acids

In a study published in the *British Medical Journal,* French researchers reported that there is a significantly lower risk of developing Alzheimer's disease among older people who eat fish at least once a week. "There is an inverse relationship between the frequency of fish consumption and the incidence of dementia," according to the lead author, Dr. Pascale Barberger-Gateau. Older people who ate fish at least once a week had about a 33 percent decrease in dementia risk over seven years. Dr. Barberger-Gateau and colleagues evaluated fish, seafood, and meat consumption among 1,674 normal aging individuals over 67 years old living in southwestern France. Over the seven years of follow-up, they found that increased fish and seafood consumption significantly reduced the chance of developing dementia.

While there are many myths and misconceptions about dietary fat, some fat is essential. Your brain is 60 percent fat. The 100 billion nerve cells in the cerebral cortex of your brain require essential fatty acids to function. Low cholesterol levels can cause depression or anger and sometimes suicide or homicide. A few of the processes that cholesterol is required for are

- Proper functioning of nerves
- Integrity of the outer membranes of all cells
- Steroid hormone formation
- Production of bile acids for digestion

There are two main categories of fat—good fat (the unsaturated kind) and bad fat (the saturated kind). Saturated fats are molecules whose binding sites are literally saturated with hydrogen. Saturated fats are very stiff and contribute to hardening of the arteries and cholesterol plaques. Saturated fats are found in meat, eggs, and dairy foods (like butter and milk) and don't spoil as easily as their healthier counterparts, the unsaturated fats.

The binding sites of unsaturated fats (mono- or polyunsaturated) are not fully saturated by hydrogen and are more flexible, which is why unsaturated fats melt at a lower temperature than saturated fats. These fats rot more easily when exposed to air, metabolize more easily, and lower blood cholesterol levels. Monounsaturated fats lower LDL cholesterol, which makes a major contribution to hardening your arteries. Monounsaturated fats also raise HDL cholesterol, which protects against cardiovascular disease. While polyunsaturated fats also provide the beneficial effect of lowering LDL cholesterol, they also lower HDL cholesterol, which is not good. The monounsaturated fats are therefore better than the polyunsaturated fats. Monounsaturated fats are found in avocados, nuts (such as almonds, cashews, and pistachio nuts), canola oil, olive oil, and peanut oil. Polyunsaturated fats are found in safflower oil, corn oil, and some fish.

The polyunsaturated fats found in salmon and mackerel and the monounsaturated fats found in canola oil and soybean oil are high in essential fatty acids (EFAs), called omega-3 fatty acids. These cannot be synthesized by the human body and therefore must be in our diet (hence the name essential fatty acids). Omega-3 fatty acids are considered good fat because they are important components of our cells and cell membranes that are essential for life and health.

It is hard to get enough omega-3 fatty acids in our diet. The foods that are now considered "mainstream" are often deficient in omega-3. Even if your diet includes several meals of fish per week, you may not be ingesting sufficient amounts of omega-3. This is because much of the fish we consume is now farm-raised or does not contain significant amounts of omega-3. When ordering fish in a restaurant or buying it at the store, ask if it was caught in the wild or farm raised. Ideally, your diet should supply at least 650 mg of long-chain omega-3 (DHA + EPA) per day, either from food sources or dietary supplementation. Omega-3 fatty acids are found in deep-sea cold-water fish such as salmon, mackerel, and sardines. Omega-6 fatty acids are also important but are usually found in adequate amounts in corn, safflower, sunflower, or soybean oils.

Flaxseed oil is not as good a source of omega-3, because your body has to convert its omega-3 fatty acid (alpha-linolenic acid) to docosahexaenoic acid (DHA). This conversion can be inefficient. Fish, however, do the work for us by converting omega-3 to DHA and eicosapentaenoic acid (EPA). You can therefore eat less fish than flaxseed oil and still get what your body needs.

Heart disease was the first area investigated with regard to the health impact of omega-3 fatty acids. It was noticed in the early 1970s that the Inuit people of Greenland had a high-fat, high-cholesterol diet yet had healthy hearts. Subsequent investigations concluded that this was due to the high level of omega-3 fatty acids in their native diet of fish and marine animals. Since then, several other studies, including two large American studies in 1997 and 1998, have revealed the same thing: that cardiovascular health is enhanced among weekly fish eaters when compared with those who ate fish only infrequently.

Omega-3 may help increase the flexibility of the red blood cell membranes, making the blood less sludgy and more fluid. This helps maintain healthy circulation everywhere in the body, including the brain. Numerous studies have found that a diet that includes a weekly serving of fish, especially those rich in omega-3, provides a health benefit to the heart and cardiovascular system. And even a diet that includes only one fish serving per week has been shown to provide this benefit. In a 1998 study of 20,551 male physicians aged 40 to 84 years, published in the *Journal of the American Medical Association,* it was found that eating fish at least once a week helped to maintain a healthy heart and cardiovascular system, compared with those who only ate fish less than once a month. The strongest confirmation has come from the publication of three randomized clinical trials, all of which reported benefits to patients with preexisting coronary artery disease. The most convincing of these was an Italian study in which 5,654 patients with coronary artery disease were randomized to either omega-3 fatty acids (850 mg/day) or the usual care. After three and a half years, those taking the omega-3 fatty acids had experienced a 20 percent reduction in overall mortality and a 45 percent decrease in risk for sudden cardiac death. These findings support the view that relatively small intakes of omega-3 fatty acids help protect heart function.

We've all heard fish called brain food. In fact, the most polyunsaturated of the omega-3 fatty acids (DHA) makes up a large portion of the gray matter of the brain. The fat in your brain is the type that forms cell membranes and plays a vital role in how our cells function. Neurons are also rich in omega-3 fatty acids. In fact, there's more DHA in our neurons than in our red blood cells; it is also found in high quantities in the retina, the light-sensitive part of the eye.

Research in the last few years has revealed that diets rich in omega-3 fatty acids may help promote a healthy emotional balance and positive mood in later years, possibly because DHA is a main component of the brain's synapses. A Danish team of researchers compared the diets of 5,386 healthy older individuals and found that the more fish in a person's diet, the longer the person was able to maintain a normal mental status.

Finally, Dr. J. A. Conquer and his colleagues from the University of Guelph in Ontario, Canada, studied the blood fatty acid content in mild cognitive impairment and dementia (62). She noted that DHA levels were low in all forms of mild cognitive impairment and dementia.

Good Fats (High in Omega-3)	Bad Fats (High in Omega-6)
Anchovies	Bacon
Avocados	Butter
Brazil nuts	Cheese (regular fat)
Canola oil	Cream sauces
Cashews	Doughnuts
Flaxseed oil	Fried foods, such as potatoes/onion
Green leafy vegetables	rings
Herring	Ice cream
Lean meats	Lamb chops
Olive oil	Mackerel
Peanut oil	Margarine
Pistachio nuts	Potato chips (fried)
Salmon	Processed foods
Sardines	Steak
Soybean oil	Whole milk
Trout	
Tuna	
Walnuts	
Whitefish	

Given the recent data on the healthful effects of eating fish and omega-3 fatty acids, we think it is reasonable to increase the amount of fish in your diet or take a daily fish oil, omega-3–fatty acid supplement. Dr. Amen has several favorite sources of fish oil supplementation. The first is a fish oil supplement called Coromega. It is made by European Reference Botanical Laboratories (ERBL; go to www.coromega.com for information). Coromega is a high-quality supplement that gives the right ratio of EPA to DHA, and it tastes great. Often fish oil supplements leave a fishy taste, but Coromega tastes like orange pudding, and we can even get children to take it without a fuss. And Dr. Rene Thomas has made an incredible-tasting, healthy ice cream, called Nature's Mighty Bites (www.kidsneedusnow.org) that contains high doses of omega-3 fatty acids. The wonderful thing is that the ice cream also contains high levels of high-quality protein and is not filled with empty calories. Life is good when you can get your fish oil supplement in orange pudding or ice cream. Dr. Barry Sears also makes a very high-quality fish oil, which can be found at www.searslabs.com. Nordic Naturals and Omega Brite, as well, make high-quality fish oil products.

Dietary Antioxidants

Dietary intake of antioxidants from fruits and vegetables reduces the risk of developing Alzheimer's disease by about 20 percent (5). Foods containing vitamin C were only effective when they were eaten with foods containing vitamin E. While dietary sources of antioxidants are probably more optimal than supplements, at least one well-designed study of vitamin supplements has also shown preventive effects for memory (63). This three-year longitudinal study of 2,889 community residents 65–102 years old examined the effects of dietary or supplemental intake of vitamins C, E, and beta carotene on working memory, short-term memory, overall mental skill, and complex task performance. Vitamin E, in doses of 400 i.u. per day or higher, reduced the rate of cognitive decline by 36 percent, compared to subjects taking the lowest amount of vitamin E. Vitamin C and beta carotene taken separately showed no effect. This is the first clinical trial evidence that supplemental vitamin E delays the onset of decline in mental skills in normal aging individuals.

The studies were conducted because it has been thought that free-radical formation has a role in the development of Alzheimer's disease. When a cell converts oxygen into energy, tiny molecules called free radicals are made. When produced in normal amounts, free radicals work to rid the body of harmful toxins, thereby keeping it healthy. When produced in toxic amounts, however, free radicals damage the body's cellular machinery, resulting in cell death and tissue damage. This process is called oxidative stress. Several lines of evidence previously implied that free-radical damage to cell membranes could disrupt normal neuronal cell functioning, leading to the formation of BA42 plaques and to neuronal cell death. Hence it was hoped that dietary intake of antioxidants such as vitamins E and C and beta carotene might inhibit the production of free radicals. Working independently on two continents, researchers in Rotterdam, the Netherlands, and in Chicago, Illinois, found evidence to support these hypotheses.

Good sources of vitamin C are tomatoes, fruits (especially citrus and kiwi), melon, raw cabbage, green leafy vegetables, peppers, sprouts, broccoli, and cabbage. Important sources of vitamin E are grains, nuts, milk, egg yolk, wheat germ, vegetable oils, and green leafy vegetables.

Blueberries are an especially good source of antioxidants. A series of studies feeding blueberries to rats have examined effects on learning new motor skills as well as protection against stroke. Rats fed blueberries showed better learning of new motor skills as they aged compared with their study counterparts. Rats fed a blueberry-enriched diet who were then given a stroke lost only 17 percent of the neurons in their hippocampus, compared with 42 percent neuron loss in rats not eating blueberries (64).

Strawberries and spinach have also shown significant protective effects in these rat models, although not as strongly as blueberries. In addition, the rats receiving these antioxidant-enriched diets all showed increased levels of vitamin E in their brains. "The exciting finding from this study is the potential reversal of some age-related impairment in both memory and motor coordination, especially with blueberry supplements," says Molly Wagster, Ph.D., a health scientist administrator with the National Institutes of Aging, speaking at an NIMH-sponsored seminar in Rockville, Maryland.

The Best Antioxidant Fruits and Vegetables (from the U.S. Department of Agriculture)

Prunes   Plums

Raisins   Broccoli

STEPS TO PREVENTION   137

Blueberries	Beets
Blackberries	Avocados
Cranberries	Oranges
Strawberries	Red grapes
Spinach	Red bell peppers
Raspberries	Cherries
Brussels sprouts	Kiwis

Estrogen

Recommended	Yes, if hysterectomy with ovary removal or severe estradiol deficiency
	Yes, if family history of dementia in parent or sibling
	No, if high risk for breast cancer
Level of evidence	Excellent
ADRD risk reduced	Dementia if hysterectomy/severe estradiol deficiency
Amount risk reduced	50 percent
Suggested dose	Estradiol, 0.5 mg/day or less
Suggested monitoring	Annual monitoring for serum estradiol level, breast and endometrial cancer, coronary artery disease, bone density

Whether or not to recommend estrogen prevention of specific ADRD risks has become an enormously complex issue in light of recent studies that suggest that supplementing estrogen has a negative effect on health. Estrogen is a hormone produced by the ovaries. Like all hormones, estrogen optimally operates at levels that are neither too high nor too low. This is why menopause, which markedly reduces estrogen, is a difficult treatment issue for physicians. However, natural estrogen therapy during or after menopause has several definite benefits, including

- Treating the physical symptoms of menopause
- Preventing osteoporosis, which severely disables mobility in women and men
- Reducing dementia risk due to severe estradiol deficiency (hysterectomy or otherwise)

The beneficial effects of estrogen on brain function are numerous and come from both basic and clinical research. These effects include

- Improved language and working memory
- Helping new synapse formation
- Increasing brain blood flow
- Enhancing nerve growth factor, which regulates acetylcholine neuron function
- 17-beta-estradiol protects neurons from free-radical damage and programmed cell death
- Reducing inflammation in the brain

However, not all studies have shown beneficial effects of estrogen in preventing or treating AD. Some of the factors that can explain the differing conclusions of these studies include: (1) the form of estrogen (Premarin is the most common form of synthetic estrogen prescribed, estradiol is the most common natural estrogen, and Evista is the most common selective estrogen receptor modulator); (2) when treatment is started (it seems that estrogen doesn't help to start once Alzheimer's is present); (3) treatment duration; (4) whether estrogen is given with or without progesterone; and (5) differences in the genetic risks for coronary heart disease and AD.

Even though the recent studies on estrogen-related health risks were well designed, there is a fundamental issue that needs to be understood when you hear news reports about their negative findings. Premarin, the form of estrogen taken by 90 percent of the women, does not reduce AD risk and is ineffective in treating women with AD. However, estradiol in low doses of 0.5 mg per day or less provides a modest treatment benefit in AD women. Furthermore, severe estradiol deficiency due to hysterectomy without subsequent estrogen replacement doubles the risk of becoming demented. So unless the different forms of estrogen are analyzed separately, you can only conclude that the findings apply to Premarin, not estradiol or Evista.

Unfortunately, the recent negative studies did not separately analyze Premarin, estradiol, and Evista when they reported the following risks for women taking estrogen after menopause for more than five years. These risks therefore only apply to Premarin until proven otherwise. The risks of taking Premarin or Prempro are (65)

- 1.3 times greater risk of heart disease (coronary artery disease)
- 1.2 times greater risk of stroke due to blood clotting but not hardening of the arteries
- 2.1 times greater risk of stroke in veins (slow-flowing blood)
- 1.8 times greater risk of gallbladder stones
- A higher risk of endometrial cancer that is eliminated by taking progestin with estrogen
- A breast cancer risk that increases with increasing estrogen levels
- 1.25 times lower risk of colon cancer
- A much lower risk of osteoporosis (also obtained with Evista)
- An unclear effect on the risk of dementia

The mental effects of severe estradiol deficiency due to hysterectomy with ovary removal have only been examined in a small case-control study from Egypt (66). Estradiol deficiency markedly impaired attention span (working memory), visual short-term memory, and the ability to remember short stories. Using electrical measurements, the researchers also found that the neurons in the estradiol-deficient women transmitted electrical signals much more slowly than in women with normal estradiol levels.

The effect of estradiol level on breast cancer has also been studied (67). Japanese women who survived the atomic bomb in 1945 had serum estradiol levels taken in 1970 and are being monitored throughout their lives for various diseases. The study found that the risk of breast cancer in 2000 increased—from 1.0 to a maximum of 3.4 times the risk of women with the lowest free-estradiol levels—as free-estradiol levels increased. Women who take estradiol should try to keep the free estradiol serum levels below the 60th percentile to minimize the risk of breast cancer.

In conclusion, it is clear that whether or not to take estrogen after menopause is a complex issue. However, the following recommendations can be gleaned from the scientific literature:

- Premarin should not be used for estrogen replacement after meno-pause.
- Low-dose estradiol (0.5 mg/day or less) is a much safer alternative.
- Evista or Fosamax are safe alternatives for treating osteoporosis, but their effect on dementia risk is not studied.
- Women with a high risk of colon cancer or dementia or who have had a hysterectomy, including ovary removal, are more likely to reduce relevant risks by taking low-dose estradiol after menopause.
- Women with low risks for stroke and breast cancer can more safely take low-dose estradiol.
- Women with high risks for breast cancer, stroke, or gallbladder stones should probably not take low-dose estradiol at this time until more data are available but can take Evista if necessary.
- Women taking estrogen after menopause need to be monitored by their physicians annually.

Exercise

Recommended	Yes, unless there is a good reason not to
Level of evidence	Excellent
ADRD risk reduced	Depression, cognitive impairment, dementia, AD, VD, coronary heart disease, stroke, high cholesterol, diabetes, high blood pressure, osteoporosis, obesity, colon and breast cancer
Amount risk reduced	ADRD 50 percent
Suggested dose	Resistive and endurance exercise, 30 minutes or more per session, three or more times per week, but preferably daily
Suggested monitoring	Annual monitoring for coronary artery disease, bone density, fasting lipid panel, fasting glucose, high blood pressure, weight

Exercise protects you from illnesses of aging. In a large study in Quebec, Dr. Danielle Laurin and her colleagues explored the association between physical activity and the risk of cognitive impairment and dementia (18). They gathered information from a community sample of 9,008 randomly selected men and women 65 years or older, who were evaluated in the 1991–1992 Canadian Study of Health and Aging, a prospective group study of dementia. Of the 6,434 eligible subjects who were cognitively normal at baseline, 4,615 completed a five-year follow-up. Screening and clinical evaluations were done at both times of the study. In 1996–1997, 3,894 remained without cognitive impairment, 436 were diagnosed as having cognitive impairment but no dementia (mild cognitive impairment), and 285 were diagnosed as having dementia. Compared with no exercise, physical activity was associated with lower risks of cognitive impairment, Alzheimer's disease, and dementia of any type. Exercise was found to be helpful in protecting against ADRD. High levels of physical activity were associated with even more reduced risks. The researchers concluded that regular physical activity could represent an important and potent protective factor for cognitive decline and dementia in elderly people.

The best kind of exercise improves the pump force of your heart (cardiovascular exercise) and strengthens the muscles of your body (resistive exercise). Cardiovascular exercise involves gradually warming up your muscles, then exercising them for 30 minutes or more to develop muscle tone for endurance (e.g., walking, running, swimming, rowing, cycling, stair climbing, cross-country skiing, etc.). Resistive exercise builds muscles' strength by exercising them against resistance (situps, pushups, lifting weights, rowing, stair climbing, swimming, cycling, cross-country skiing, and so on). As you can see, several types of exercise fall into both categories, including rowing, stair climbing, swimming, cycling, and cross-country skiing. You can also make walking and running resistive exercises if you add weights, carry your infant, your dog, or your mate!

Exercise exerts a protective effect on hippocampal neurons that lasts about three days. Therefore, the minimum frequency of exercise is every three days, or three times a week. Studies have shown that the more frequently you exercise, the greater the benefits.

Exercise also enhances the production of glutathione, which is the major antioxidant in all cells, to protect your muscles and other tissues against free radical damage. However, chronic inactivity ("couch potato" syndrome) reduces cell glutathione levels so that free radicals can damage your cells and trigger programmed cell death.

Exercise also increases the chemical nitric oxide, which helps keep blood vessel walls open and round. In order to keep your blood vessels open, blood needs to pulse through them. Without good blood flow, the levels of nitric oxide drop and cause the blood vessel walls to become distorted and limit the flow of blood. The most effective way to make blood flow pulse through arteries is to exercise. Without pulsatile flow, the blood vessels in the deep areas of the brain distort, block blood flow, and cause the accumulation of tiny strokes. Over a period of years, these strokes accumulate and cause these deep brain areas to stop working. The deep areas of the brain control leg movement, coordinated body movement, and speed of thinking and behaving. Strokes in these areas produce a clinical picture that closely resembles Parkinson's disease because it affects similar brain areas. This is why people who do not exercise after 40 years old are not as mentally sharp as people who regularly exercise.

The benefits of mild to moderate exercise, if you are over 40 years old, include (23)

- Protecting brain cells against toxins, including free radicals and excess glutamate
- Repairing your DNA to help protect against programmed cell death
- Reducing the risks of cognitive impairment and dementia due to AD and related disorders in persons over 65 years old by about 50 percent
- Preserving your mental abilities after age 70
- Reducing risks of heart disease and stroke by improving cholesterol and fat metabolism, plus improving blood, oxygen, and glucose delivery to tissues
- Reducing risk of diabetes by making insulin better control your blood sugar (glucose), and increasing your lean-to-fat mass ratio
- Reducing risk of osteoporosis by reducing bone loss (estrogen enhances this effect)
- Reducing risk of depression
- Reducing risks of colon and breast cancer
- Reducing risks of falling by improving muscle tone and endurance, and reducing strokes to the deep brain areas

Ginkgo Biloba

Recommended	Yes, in the presence of ADRD risk factors •
Level of evidence	Excellent
ADRD risk reduced	Cholesterol, coronary artery disease, high blood pressure, stroke
Amount risk reduced	Not known
Suggested dose	60–120 mg twice a day
Suggested monitoring	None

Ginkgo biloba, from the Chinese ginkgo tree, is a powerful antioxidant that is best known for its ability to enhance circulation. The best-studied form of ginkgo biloba is a special extract called EBG 761, which has been studied in blood vessel disease, clotting disorders, depression, and Alzheimer's disease. A comparison in 2000 of all the published, placebo-controlled studies longer than six months for ginkgo biloba extract, EGB 761, versus Cognex, Aricept, and Exelon showed they all had similar benefits for mild to moderate AD patients (68). Ginkgo biloba is most frequently marketed incorrectly as a memory-enhancing supplement, which it usually is not. Its primary benefits have been shown in both animal and human studies. An animal model of rats genetically engineered to have high blood pressure showed that when fed EGB 761, they have less damage to their DNA, they have less free-radical production, and their blood vessels produce more nitric oxide to keep their blood vessel walls nice and round, which keeps blood pressure down, improves blood flow, and reduces stroke risk (69).

The most widely publicized study in the United States of ginkgo biloba was done by Dr. P. L. Le Bars and his colleagues at the New York Institute for Medical Research, and it appeared in the *Journal of the American Medical Association* in 1997 (6). In this study EGB 761 was used to assess the efficacy and safety in treating Alzheimer's disease and vascular dementia. It was a 52-week multicenter study with patients who had mild to severe symptoms. Patients were randomly assigned to treatment with EGB 761 (120 mg/day) or placebo. Progress was monitored at 12, 26, and

52 weeks; 202 patients finished the study. At the end of the study the authors concluded that EGB is safe and appears to be capable of stabilizing and, in a substantial number of cases, improving the cognitive performance and the social functioning of demented patients for six months to one year. Although modest, the changes induced by EGB were objectively measured and were of sufficient magnitude to be recognized by the caregivers.

There are many different forms of ginkgo, making dosing confusing. In the United States Gingkoba and Ginkgold (Nature's Way) are brands that have been compounded to reflect high-quality EGB 761. The usual effective dose is 60 to 120 mg twice a day. There is a small risk of bleeding, and the dosages of other blood-thinning agents being taken may sometimes need to be reduced.

Human Growth Hormone (HGH)

Recommended	No
Level of evidence	Poor
ADRD risk reduced	None
Amount risk reduced	N/A
Suggested dose	N/A

Like all hormones, human growth hormone (HGH) has its place in medicine. It can improve muscle strength and energy in the severely debilitated. Too much HGH leads to apathy, reduced sex drive, dejection, brooding, irritability, increased appetite, poor concentration, and fatigue. There is no indication that it improves mental abilities other than through its effects on energy. It has not been shown to be useful as a preventive agent for any ADRD risk factor and may actually increase risk of AD, heart disease, stroke, and atherosclerosis.

Melatonin

Recommended	Yes, if there are sleep problems
Level of evidence	Fair
ADRD risk reduced	Not yet defined
Amount risk reduced	Not yet defined
Suggested dose	0.3 mg to 3 mg
Suggested monitoring	None

A number of studies have documented disturbances in the sleep-wake pattern (circadian rhythm) associated with Alzheimer's disease, resulting in changes of body temperature, hormonal concentrations, sleep-wake patterns, and rest-activity cycles. These cycles are regulated by the daily rise and fall of melatonin levels. One of the symptoms associated with the aging process has been a decline in the amplitude of the melatonin rhythm; subsequently there is currently interest in using melatonin to treat sleep disturbances in Alzheimer's disease. Experiments with melatonin have been shown to reduce oxidative damage to nuclear DNA. A variety of studies also suggest that melatonin may inhibit BA42 toxicity. Some researchers hypothesize that an age-related decline in melatonin could be a cause of Alzheimer's disease, but it is just as probable that the disruption of the melatonin cycle is the result of an underlying disease process. The usual dose is 3 mg, but some research indicates lower doses (0.3 mg) are effective and 3 mg may result in disrupted sleep for some. We think that melatonin is worth a try if you are having trouble sleeping, but be aware that you may need to adjust your dose.

Mental Exercise

Recommended	Yes
Level of evidence	Excellent
ADRD risk reduced	AD, cognitive impairment, dementia
Amount risk reduced	AD 33 percent, cognitive impairment 47 percent
Suggested dose	Daily, 1 hour or more
Suggested monitoring	None

Lifelong learning and mental exercise are essential to keeping your brain healthy for as long as possible. The now famous "Nun Study" is perhaps the best example of how mental activity can prevent cognitive impairment or AD (70). In this study, 801 normal elderly Catholic nuns, priests, and brothers were recruited from 40 groups across the United States. After four and a half years, 111 (14 percent) had developed AD. Researchers at the Rush Alzheimer's Center in Chicago examined the influence of common cognitive activities, such as reading a newspaper, by creating a five-point Cognitive Activity Frequency Scale. After controlling for factors that could confuse the results, such as age, sex, education, and baseline intelligence, they found that a one-point (20 percent) increase in cognitive activity score reduced AD risk by 33 percent, reduced decline in global cognition by 47 percent, reduced working memory decline by 60 percent, and reduced slowing of perceptual speed by 30 percent.

What Kinds of Mental Exercise Are Helpful?

Almost any mental activity you enjoy can be used to protect your brain from AD. The essential requirement of the mental activity is that it activate a wide variety of brain areas, one of which must be the hippocampus and entorhinal cortex (in the temporal lobes), which stores new learning for retrieval later on. By using your hippocampus and entorhinal cortex, you are protecting the first brain area affected by AD. In essence, as long as you learn something new about your favorite mental activity, and try to recall it later, you are protecting short-term memory from the ravages of AD and other causes of dementia.

When you read, you learn something new (encoding) and attempt to recall it later (retrieval). Reading activates:

- The occipital, temporal, and parietal lobes to process and interpret what you read (perception)
- The midfrontal lobes to follow and understand the material (understanding)
- The tips of the frontal lobes to analyze the material (analysis)
- The midfrontal lobes to retrieve relevant information already stored in your brain (retrieval)

- The tips of the frontal lobes to make any necessary decisions (execution)
- The entorhinal cortex and hippocampus to store what you want to recall later (learning)

Reading stimulates a wide variety of brain areas that process, understand, and analyze what you read, then store it for later recall if you decide it's worth remembering. The neurons in these activated brain areas are repetitively stimulated with specific patterns of information, which cause the synapses of these neurons to be strengthened by long-term potentiation (LTP; see Chapter 2, page 18). Each time you read, the neurons activated in your brain's visual circuits further strengthen their synapses so you can process what you read with increasing efficiency. Each time you try to understand what you read, the neurons in your working memory circuits strengthen their synapses so you can understand reading material with increasing efficiency. Each time you try to learn something you read for recall later, the neurons in the hippocampus and entorhinal cortex further strengthen their synapses so you can encode and store new information with increasing efficiency. Each time you try to recall what you just learned, after a delay of at least two minutes, neurons in the frontal lobe further strengthen their synapses so you can retrieve stored information with increasing efficiency.

Each component of a mental activity shares a common process that leads to repetitive activation of neurons and synapses in the brain circuits used, followed by greater efficiency. This is why moderately to severely demented persons can still perform their best-learned skills or abilities after they have lost those that were less frequently used. A memorable example occurred with one of Dr. Shankle's AD patients, a professional jazz pianist, who continued performing at nightclubs even though he could no longer read music or say his name!

Crossword puzzles require reading (perception), understanding the hint (understanding), analyzing the hint (analysis), searching your brain and retrieving possible answers (retrieval), and deciding which answer is correct (execution). If you try to remember something you learned while doing the crossword puzzle and try to retrieve it later (after at least two minutes' delay), then crossword puzzles also activate your hippocampus and entorhinal cortex.

Writing is a mental activity in which the input comes from your brain instead of the outside world. However, the words, sounds, and images that make up what you wish to write down are activated by the same brain areas as those that would be activated if the this information were coming from the outside world (perception). Your frontal lobes interpret these perceptions (understanding), analyze them in the context of what you wish to express (analysis), search your brain to retrieve other relevant information (retrieval), decide what to write, then write it (execution). Should you learn something interesting in the process of writing, decide to remember it, and try to recall it later, then writing also activates your hippocampus and entorhinal cortex (learning).

Active Versus Passive Television Watching

While studies have shown that excessive TV watching is fundamentally bad for you, it is quite possible that the way you watch TV is more important than TV watching itself. When you watch TV, your eyes and ears are engaged to activate visual and auditory brain circuits (perception). As with reading, crossword puzzles, and writing, your frontal lobes process this information (perception), interpret it (understanding), analyze it in the context of the situation (analysis), and search your brain to retrieve related information (retrieval). Up to this point, TV watching is mostly a passive, automatic activity that takes little effort. However, if you have a reason for watching a particular TV program other than simply relaxing, your frontal lobes will evaluate what to do with the information (execution), and your hippocampus and entorhinal cortex will store it to be used later (learning). These last two parts are what we call active TV watching. Watching a soap opera, ball game, or movie is likely to be passive TV watching. However, watching the Discovery channel to learn how Tutankhamen was mummified, watching the Food channel to learn how to make a new recipe, or watching the History channel to learn about Franklin Delano Roosevelt are all examples of active TV watching, which may very well protect your brain from AD in the same ways that reading, writing, and other cognitive activities do.

How you engage in a mental activity may be more important than the type of mental activity itself, so TV watching—if an active process—may protect your brain from AD.

Nonsteroidal Anti-inflammatory Medications (NSAIDs)

Recommended	Yes, if well tolerated
Level of evidence	Excellent
ADRD risk reduced	AD, heart attack, stroke, peripheral vascular disease
Amount risk reduced	50 percent
Suggested dose	200 mg a day ibuprofen or equivalent
Suggested monitoring	Annual stool sample to check for bleeding, kidney tests, possibly serum beta amyloid once commercially available

Nine out of ten population-based studies have shown that NSAIDs used in low doses for two or more years in persons under 80 years old reduce the chance of developing AD by about 50 percent (59). Some of these studies have shown also that the risk reduction occurs with low-dose NSAIDs (less than 175 mg aspirin or less than 500 mg naproxen or equivalent dose with other NSAIDs). Information from the well-designed Baltimore Longitudinal Study of Aging showed that the risk-reducing effect of NSAIDs began after taking them for two or more years.

NSAIDs and Mild Cognitive Impairment

Mild cognitive impairment is now thought to be an early symptomatic stage of AD and other dementing disorders in many individuals. Data from another large study showed that persons taking low to moderate doses of NSAIDs performed better on cognitive screening tests than people not taking NSAIDs or taking high doses of NSAIDs.

How NSAIDs Reduce AD Risk

Contrary to initial thinking, reducing inflammation does not appear to be the mechanism of the risk reduction effect on AD. Low doses of NSAIDs appear to inhibit the production of beta amyloid, which is thought to be one of the three primary mechanisms of damage caused by AD. To date, only three NSAIDs have been found to reduce beta amyloid formation (47): (1) ibuprofen (i.e., Motrin, Advil); (2) clinoril (Sulindac); and (3) indomethacin (Indocin). At present, none of the "stomach-protective" NSAIDs—including Vioxx, Mobic, and Celebrex—have been shown to reduce risk of AD.

Why All NSAIDs Don't Delay AD Once Symptoms Have Developed

Until recently, it was unclear why NSAIDs delay the onset but not the progression of AD once symptoms have developed. A study in genetically engineered mice who develop the neuritic plaques of AD may explain this enigma. Paul T. Jantzen and his colleagues examined the effects of the NSAIDs NCX-2216, flurbiprofen, ibuprofen, and Celebrex (71). NCX-2216 is similar to flurbiprofen but stimulates nitric oxide release (the same chemical that helps keep blood vessels open). The genetically engineered "AD" mice were fed a diet that included either NCX-2216, flurbiprofen, ibuprofen, or Celebrex between the ages of 7 and 12 months. When the researchers looked at the brains of these mice, they found that only NCX-2216 markedly reduced the form of beta amyloid that is found in toxic neuritic plaques of AD. Only NCX-2216 activated certain brain cells to clear beta amyloid from neuritic plaques. This inability of some NSAIDs to reduce the load of beta amyloid in the neuritic plaques of "AD" mice would explain why some NSAIDs do not work once neuritic plaques have formed and AD symptoms appear. These findings determined that nitric oxide helps activate certain brain cells to clear beta amyloid from neuritic plaques. The development of NSAIDs like NCX-2216 could provide a new way to prevent AD by delaying both its onset and progression.

At present, given that some NSAIDs block beta amyloid formation and others do not, it appears that the ones most likely to reduce AD risk are ibuprofen, clinoril, and indomethacin. Ibuprofen is available over the counter. Clinoril is prescription and is also relatively safe, while indomethacin is associated with more frequent side effects. Low doses of ibuprofen and clinoril are 200 mg and 50–100 mg once a day respectively. These NSAIDs should be taken with meals to reduce stomach irritation and the likelihood of gastrointestinal bleeding. The AD risk reduction of about 50 percent begins after at least two years of use.

The following tests should be monitored by your physician, if you are taking NSAIDs or aspirin, to minimize the chance of complications due to gastrointestinal bleeding, ulcers, and reduced kidney function: a stool blood test and kidney screening tests.

Phosphatidylserine (PS)

Recommended	Yes, if well tolerated
Level of evidence	Excellent
ADRD risk reduced	Memory decline
Amount risk reduced	Not yet known
Suggested dose	100 mg three times a day
Suggested monitoring	None

A naturally occurring nutrient that is found in foods such as fish, green leafy vegetables, soy products and rice, PS is a component of cell membranes that works with another molecule, diacylglycerol, to help maintain the cell's internal activity via protein kinase C (72).

Despite reports of the potential of PS to help improve age-related declines in memory, learning, verbal skills, and concentration, its value in treating AD and other causes of cognitive impairment is largely untested in well-defined disease groups. Studies using PET scans of AD patients who have taken PS show that it produces a general increase in metabolic activity in the brain, which is consistent with its known cellular function. However, unlike the approved treatments for AD, PS does not electively improve the activity of brain areas that are impaired in AD persons (73).

Although there are relatively few double-blind, placebo-controlled studies using PS to treat AD or any other specific disease causing dementia, a number of studies have used PS in treating cognitive impairment or dementia. Since cognitive impairment and dementia are not themselves diseases but rather combinations of symptoms, it is not clear what PS is treating other than symptoms. With this cautionary note in mind, PS may be useful in treating some of the symptoms of cognitive impairment or dementia. Effective doses of PS have been reported to be 300 mg per day.

The types of symptoms that have improved in placebo-controlled studies of cognitive impairment or dementia include loss of interest, reduced activities, social isolation, anxiety, and loss of memory, concentration, and recall. Milder stages of impairment tend to respond to PS better than more severe stages.

With regard to depression in elderly individuals, Dr. M. Maggioni and his colleagues studied the effects of oral PS (300 mg/day) versus placebo, and noted significant improvements in mood, memory, and motivation after 30 days of PS treatment.

Statins

Recommended	Take statins if high cholesterol is present
Level of evidence	Good
ADRD risk reduced	High cholesterol, heart attack, stroke
Amount risk reduced	50–79 percent for ADRD
Suggested dose	Varies for each type
Suggested monitoring	Cholesterol levels, liver enzymes

Statins are a class of drugs that lower cholesterol. They are derived from red rice yeast extract, which blocks the synthesis of cholesterol in the liver. Common statins include Mevacor (lovastatin), Zocor (simvastatin), Pravachol (pravastatin), Lescol (fluvastatin), and Lipitor (atorvastatin). Statin drugs have an impact on blood vessels in the brain, and recent studies suggest that statins can significantly reduce the risk of stroke, a risk factor for AD. They may also potentially be involved in preventing Alzheimer's disease and other types of dementia.

The largest study conducted to date examining the association between statin use and risk of Alzheimer's disease was done by researchers at Boston University School of Medicine. They compared the risk factors and medication history in 912 individuals with probable or definite Alzheimer's disease and in 1,669 of their family members who did not have dementia. After adjusting for a number of factors, including age, sex, ethnicity, and apoE gene status, they discovered that study subjects who took statin drugs had a 79 percent reduction in Alzheimer's disease risk, irrespective of race or apoE gene status. Other cholesterol-lowering drugs showed a trend toward lower risk for Alzheimer's disease, but the results were not statistically significant. Further support of this protective effect of statins came from the Canadian Health Study of the Aging (42), in which 492 Canadians over 65 years old developed dementia after their initial assessment, and were compared with 823 persons who remained normal. The researchers found that the risk for developing AD among statin users was 74 percent lower than for those who did not use statins. The only group that did not show this benefit were subjects over 80 years old.

Researchers in Holland studied 561 patients aged 85 years and found that those with the lowest levels of HDL cholesterol (good cholesterol) were more than twice as likely to have dementia as those with higher levels. After excluding patients with documented heart disease or stroke, the increased risk of dementia with low HDL levels became even more apparent; HDL may prevent the formation of plaques associated with dementia or may reduce inflammation in the brain.

Several other well-designed studies in people with high cholesterol now show that statins reduce the risk for developing memory loss or other impairments in mental skills due to ADRD by twofold to fourfold. The basis for the reduced AD risk may be the ability of statins to block the formation of beta amyloid in neurons. One study of nondemented people with elevated LDL showed that Lipitor (atorvastatin) in doses from 40 to 60 mg a day, but not less than 40 mg daily, lowered blood levels of beta amyloid compared with placebo. Another study of Zocor (simvastatin), 80 mg daily in 44 AD patients, showed that levels of the 40-amino-acid form of beta amyloid were reduced in the cerebrospinal fluid in the less severe AD patients.

Red rice yeast extract actually contains lovastatin, which is marketed under the name Mevacor. If lovastatin is found to reduce beta amyloid, then so will red rice yeast extract. Therefore, red rice yeast extract may reduce AD risk in a manner similar to other statins. If so, then it is an inexpensive alternative (a one-month supply costs about $15) to the more expensive prescription statins. The usual dose of red rice yeast extract is 2,400 mg per day. It comes in 600 mg capsules and can be taken at bedtime if well tolerated (that's when the liver synthesizes most of your cholesterol) or two capsules after dinner and two capsules at bedtime. A fasting lipid panel should be checked after one month and the dose adjusted to obtain the desired cholesterol levels. You can purchase red rice yeast extract through Lifelink Nutritional Supplements at www.lifelinknet.com.

If your risk for AD is increased and you have elevated cholesterol, it may be wise to take a statin drug or red rice yeast extract to reduce both risk of heart disease from high cholesterol and risk of AD.

Vinpocetine

Recommended	Probably
Level of evidence	Good
ADRD risk reduced	AD, heart attack, stroke
Amount risk reduced	Not known
Suggested dose	10 mg three times a day
Suggested monitoring	None

Vinpocetine is derived from an extract of the common periwinkle plant (*Vinca minor*). It is a cerebral vasodilator, meaning it selectively widens arteries and capillaries, increasing blood flow to the brain. It also combats accumulation of platelets in the blood, improving circulation. Because of these properties, vinpocetine was first used in the treatment of cerebrovascular disorders and acute memory loss due to late-life dementia. It also may have a beneficial effect on memory problems associated with normal aging.

A 1976 study found that vinpocetine immediately increased circulation in 50 people with abnormal blood flow. After one month of taking moderate doses of vinpocetine, patients showed improvement on memorization tests. After a prolonged period of vinpocetine treatment, cognitive impairment diminished significantly or disappeared altogether in many of the patients. A 1987 study of elderly patients with chronic cerebral dysfunction found that patients who took vinpocetine performed better on psychological evaluations after the 90-day trial period than did those who received a placebo. More recent studies have shown that vinpocetine reduces neural damage and protects against oxidative damage from harmful beta amyloid buildup.

So how exactly does vinpocetine act in the body and how might it improve impaired memory function? As already mentioned, vinpocetine boosts circulation to the brain by increasing the amount of blood traveling through blood vessels in and around the brain. In addition, it is thought that vinpocetine accelerates the cells' activities in at least four other ways:

1. It speeds up the rate of production of the energy within nerve cells.
2. It increases the amount of glucose used by the nerve cells.
3. It increases the rate at which brain cells use the oxygen molecules taken from the blood.
4. It increases a number of different neurotransmitters in the brain, including norepinephrine, dopamine, acetylcholine, and serotonin. An extensive body of research implicates dopamine in working memory tasks and acetylcholine in memory and memory loss. Vinpocetine boosts the concentration of these critical neurotransmitters and may promote memory processing.

Vitamins

B Vitamins

Recommended	Yes
Level of evidence	Good
ADRD risk reduced	AD and heart attack
Amount risk reduced	Not known
Suggested dose	100 percent RDA multivitamin daily, including B vitamins
Suggested monitoring	None

B vitamins play an integral role in the functioning of the nervous system and help the brain synthesize neurotransmitters that affect mood and thinking. A balanced complex of the B vitamins is essential for energy and for balancing hormone levels. Folate and B_{12} deficiencies are well-known causes of cognitive impairment or dementia, as well as coronary heart disease (72). They can also elevate homocysteine levels, which increase risks for stroke, heart disease, and Alzheimer's disease. Patients deficient in folate can show significant improvements in memory and attention when treated with folic acid for as little as 60 days.

In addition to a direct effect, B vitamins indirectly impact mental function by altering the levels of harmful or beneficial substances in the body. For instance, elevated homocysteine (an amino acid) levels have been linked to heart disease and poorer cognitive function. A combination therapy with B vitamins—folate, vitamins B_{12} and B_6—is an effective means to reduce elevated homocysteine levels. To maintain low plasma homocysteine concentration, people should be advised to increase their consumption of eggs, green leafy vegetables, and fruits, which are rich in B vitamins.

Another study showed that less than optimal levels of vitamins B_6 and B_{12} and folic acid lead to a deficiency of S-adenosylmethionine (SAMe). This deficiency can cause depression, dementia, or a degeneration of the nerves. The typical American diet does not always provide these essential vitamins, at least not in high doses. Because B vitamins are water-soluble and excreted from the body daily, they must be replenished on a regular basis. Older people are at greater risk for vitamin deficiency because they tend to eat less of a variety of foods, although their requirements for certain vitamins, such as B_6, are actually higher. Older people may also have problems with efficient nutrient absorption from food. Even healthy older people often exhibit deficiencies in vitamin B_6, vitamin B_{12}, and folate.

B_6 supplementation has been found helpful for memory function. Dr. J. B. Deijen and his colleagues from Holland found in a study of 76 elderly men that giving vitamin B_6 versus placebo improved memory function.

Vitamin C (Ascorbic Acid)

Recommended	Yes
Level of evidence	Excellent
ADRD risk reduced	AD, heart attack, stroke
Amount risk reduced	20 percent when taken with vitamin E
Suggested dose	1,000 mg twice a day
Suggested monitoring	None

Vitamin C is only effective when given with vitamin E. In the Rotterdam 10-year epidemiologic study of 5,395 normal, aging, community-dwelling individuals 55 years and older, dietary intake, supplement intake, and mental status were measured, along with a variety of other risk factors. The findings of this 10-year study were that high dietary intake of vitamins C and E (fruits and vegetables) reduces the risk of AD by about 20 percent (5). Furthermore, vitamin C recycles vitamin E to make it more available to cells in the brain and body to protect against cell damage from free-radical formation. Side effects are rare but can occasionally cause urinary tract infections due to acidification. The recommended dose is 1,000 mg twice a day. Higher doses may increase the chances that women can have urinary tract infections.

Vitamin E (Alpha and Gamma Tocopherol)

Recommended	Yes
Level of evidence	Excellent
ADRD risk reduced	AD, heart attack, stroke
Amount risk reduced	36 percent
Suggested dose	100–200 i.u. twice a day, except in smokers
Suggested monitoring	None

A recent analysis of nineteen controlled clinical trials using vitamin E alone or with other supplements has provided additional details about the usefulness of vitamin E in increasing or decreasing the risks of specific diseases (87). The media presented these results as if any vitamin E dose greater than two hundred international units (i.u.) was harmful. However, a close look at the published study leads to a different conclusion. What is clear from this study is that the effective dose of vitamin E for reducing the risk of a given disease varies.

The controlled trials that showed vitamin E lowered the risk of death due to any cause included studies examining the risk of heart attack, colon cancer, esophageal dysphagia (gastritis, heartburn), progression of Alzheimer's disease, decline in nursing home patients, and the general

Table 6.1. Prevention Agents Reviewed

Prevention Agent	Risks Reduced	Recommended to Take for the Risks It Affects?	Quality of the Prevention Evidence
Acetyl-L-Carnitine (ALC)	Heart disease, stroke	Yes	Good
Alcohol	Heart disease, stroke, dementia	Maybe, if you can limit and control intake	Excellent
Alpha lipoic acid	Diabetes, stroke, solid cancers, programmed cell death	Yes	Fair
Aspirin	AD, heart attack, stroke	Yes, if well tolerated (but should not take NSAIDs the same day)	Excellent
Cat's claw	Possibly AD	No	Test tube only
Choline/lecithin	Cognitive decline	No	Animal studies only
Coenzyme Q10 (CoQ10)	Parkinson's disease, possibly Lewy body disease	Yes	Good
DHEA	None, and may increase obesity and prostate and breast cancer	No	Poor
Diet that is calorie restricted, high in fish or fish oil, high in antioxidants	ADRD, cancer, vascular disease, diabetes	Yes	Excellent
Estrogen	AD, cognitive impairment, dementia	Maybe	Good
Exercise	Depression, cognitive impairment, dementia, AD, VD, coronary heart disease, stroke, high cholesterol, diabetes, high blood pressure, osteoporosis, obesity, colon and breast cancer	Yes	Excellent
Ginkgo biloba	Cholesterol, coronary artery disease, high blood pressure, stroke	Yes, if ADRD risk factors present	Excellent
Human growth hormone	None	No	Poor
Melatonin	Sleep problems	Maybe, if sleep problems	Poor
Mental exercise	AD	Yes	Excellent

Prevention Agent	Risks Reduced	Recommended to Take for the Risks It Affects?	Quality of the Prevention Evidence
Nonsteroidal anti-inflammatory medications (NSAIDs)	AD, heart attack, stroke, peripheral vascular disease	Yes, if well tolerated (but should not take with aspirin on the same day)	Excellent
Omega-3 fatty acids	See diet	Maybe, especially if mood disorders present	Good
Phosphatidylserine	MCI and early AD	Yes	Excellent
Red rice yeast extract	AD and heart disease	Yes, if high cholesterol	Good
Statins	ADRD, heart attack, stroke, peripheral vascular disease	Yes, if high cholesterol	Good
Vinpocetine	AD, heart attack, stroke	Maybe	Good
Vitamin B	AD and heart attack, especially if high homocysteine levels	Yes	Good
Vitamin C (ascorbic acid)	AD (with vitamin E), heart attack, stroke	Yes	Excellent
Vitamin E (mixed tocotrienes/tocopherols	AD, heart attack, stroke	Yes	Excellent

population. Except for the Alzheimer's disease progression study, the dose of vitamin E was 440 i.u. or less.

The controlled trials that showed vitamin E increased the risk of death due to any cause studied progression of coronary artery disease in post-menopausal women or in persons with blood vessel imaging evidence of coronary artery disease, progression of cataracts in early onset individuals, progression of Parkinson's disease in young onset individuals, risk of heart disease in smokers, and healthy older adults. In all but the smoker study, the dose was at least 400 i.u. a day and usually higher.

The lesson to be learned from this analysis of many controlled trials is that you must know why you are taking vitamin E and how much to take in order to know if it is beneficial. For example, the Parkinson's disease study showed an increased overall death rate at a dose of 2000 i.u. of vitamin E daily. However, lower doses were not studied, so we simply do not know if they could help slow Parkinson's disease. Given that the overall death rate was lower in persons with a variety of medical conditions when doses of 400 i.u. or lower were used daily, it would seem prudent to limit vitamin E to 400 i.u. a day or less (d'alpha tocopherol or mixed tocopherols, but not dl-alpha tocopherol). Unfortunately, male smokers seem to be at increased risk of death when taking doses of vitamin E as low as 50 i.u. (i.u.s) daily. Also, it is not known whether persons with Alzheimer's disease can slow its progression when taking doses of vitamin E less than 2000 i.u. daily. In healthy persons under 65 years old, vitamin E doses of 33 to 200 i.u. lowers overall death rate. In healthy aging persons 65 years and older, overall death rate is lower when taking doses as low as 33 i.u. of vitamin E daily, but overall death rate increases when taking 500 i.u. daily.

Keeping these caveats about vitamin E in mind, here is what published studies have shown with regard to Alzheimer's disease and the slowing of cognitive decline in normal aging. Vitamin E at 1000 i.u. twice a day in people already with the symptoms of AD delays its *progression* by one year. With regards to *prevention* in normal aging individuals, a recent three-year longitudinal study of 2,889 community residents 65–102 years old examined the influence of dietary and supplemental intake of vitamins C, E, and beta-carotene on the course of a variety of mental skills (sixty-three). They tested working memory, short-term memory, overall mental ability and complex task performance. The study found that vitamin E, in doses of 400 i.u. daily or higher, resulted in a 36 percent reduction in rate of cognitive decline compared to subjects taking the lowest amount of vitamin E. Vitamin C and beta carotene taken separately showed no effect. This is the first clinical trial evidence that vitamin E delays the onset of decline in mental skills in normal aging individuals.

Recently, another study done in Rotterdam, Holland examined diet and risk for AD in 5395 people at least fifty-five years of age (5). After an average follow-up of six years, 197 participants developed dementia, of which 146 had Alzheimer disease. When adjustments were made for age, gender, alcohol intake, education, smoking habits, presence of carotid plaques, and use of antioxidative supplements, high intake of vitamin C and vitamin E was associated with a 20 percent lower risk of Alzheimer's disease. Among current smokers, this relationship was most pronounced. The associations did not vary by education or apolipoprotein E genotype.

Vitamin E is usually harmless when taken in doses of 400 units a day or less. It is an antioxidant that stabilizes lipid membranes in the brain and protects the brain from damage due to free radical formation in cells. It is known that antioxidant mechanisms decline with aging, so supplementation may be protective. Furthermore, taking vitamin C, such as 250 to 500 mg, with each dose of vitamin E improves the absorption of E into the brain. Although not yet tested in clinical trials, this probably improves the effect of vitamin E on delaying decline in mental skills.

Vitamin E side effects are rare. However, vitamin E may affect anticoagulation levels if on Coumadin and may affect cholesterol levels. For people who take vitamin E and also take Coumadin, should have regular laboratory studies to check for any bleeding problems. People who take vitamin E and also have high cholesterol should have their fasting lipid panel monitored about every three to six months to determine the effect of vitamin E on cholesterol.

The kind of vitamin E that you take matters. D-alpha tocopherol and mixed tocopherols, including alpha and gamma forms, are more effective antioxidants than dl-alpha tocopherol. D-Alpha tocopherol is the most common form sold in stores. Because of the relatively short duration of action of the tocopherols (2–4 hours), taking them twice a day after meals gives better cellular protection to your brain and body.

chapter 7

Finding the Right Diagnosis

While we were writing this book, a 50-year-old friend of Dr. Amen's complained about his memory. "I can't remember the names of simple things," he said. "I am in a fantasy football league and couldn't remember the name of my quarterback, even though it was Kurt Warner! It is happening all the time. It seems I can't remember anything." Fifty is not too early to have a problem, and it is certainly not too early to be checked.

Just as for diabetes, hypertension, breast cancer, and many other diseases, prevention and treatment strategies work best when done as an annual part of your routine medical exam once you reach 50 years old. We both have heard all too many times, "I would be afraid to check my memory and find out that I might have Alzheimer's disease." Of course you would be afraid; who wouldn't? But consider the consequences of your fear. Here are your three basic choices and consequences for dealing with the potential of ADRD—which one are you going to choose? Make a decision.

1. Have an annual memory checkup after age 50 years old by a memory specialist, such as a neurologist or neuropsychiatrist. If you are detected with memory loss before you even know you have a memory problem, you can potentially reverse it with treatment, prevent decline for six or more years, function perfectly well, and not burden your loved ones. This will save you $200,000 to $300,000 and give you a significantly increased quality of life.

2. Wait until your family tells you that you are asking the same question you asked five minutes ago. Getting diagnosed and treated at this stage (mild cognitive impairment) will stop the progression for three or more years but will burden your loved ones because of the problems created by your memory loss. They will have to hire someone to watch you at home because you could forget to turn off the oven, flood the bathroom, or perform any number of other dangerous behaviors. This will cost you about $200,000 and save about $100,000, compared with your third choice.

3. Have your loved ones take you to the doctor because you have become paranoid that they are out to get you or that people are coming into your home and stealing things. Getting diagnosed and treated at this stage (mild to moderate dementia) will stop disease progression for up to three years and significantly improve your paranoia and other behavioral and functional problems. However, you will severely burden your loved ones, be incapable of doing your favorite pastimes because of the severity of your dementia, and require almost constant supervision, and may very well need to be institutionalized. This will cost you about $300,000.

Although you probably have an excellent primary care doctor whom you trust, most doctors don't have the tools to detect memory changes early. A frightening statistic reported by Dr. Jeff Cummings and his colleagues at the University of California, Los Angeles, is that 95 percent of persons with ADRD are first diagnosed by their primary care doctor four or more years after symptoms first appeared; by then they are moderately demented. Another more recent study done in Honolulu found that in 46 to 70 percent of mildly to moderately demented Asians who see their primary care physician, symptoms regularly go undetected, even when the physician is directly asked whether he or she thinks the patient is demented (75)! However, it's not your doctor's fault. In Dr. Shankle's lectures to physicians throughout the United States, they all complain of not having practical tools to detect memory loss early. It is wonderful that SPECT and PET scans can detect ADRD before the brain loses tissue. When that happens, proper diagnosis and treatment can reverse memory loss. But to get a SPECT or PET scan early enough, doctors need to have a simple way to detect memory changes before they affect their patients' functioning. We hope that you will choose an annual memory checkup so that you and your doctor can work together to make reversing memory loss in ADRD a reality. See Appendix A for a reliable, effective screening tool.

Consider also that by 2008, even better treatments for Alzheimer's disease and other dementing disorders will be available. Detecting early changes now can keep you from declining so you can profit from these better future treatments.

Of all persons with memory loss, cognitive impairment, or dementia, only 60 percent have Alzheimer's disease. The remaining 40 percent often have curable conditions such as depression, alcohol or drug dependence, attention deficit disorder, vitamin deficiencies, thyroid disease, poor nutrition, and medication side effects.

Getting a Thorough Assessment

Find the Right Professional

The following health professionals may have received training in evaluating early changes in mental clarity, memory, other mental abilities, mood, behavior, or personality: (1) neurologist; (2) psychiatrist; (3) neuropsychologist; (4) geriatrician (a specialist in the care of older adults); (5) internist; (6) primary care doctor; (7) nurse practitioner; or (8) physician's assistant.

What is more important than their particular specialty is whether they are trained in evaluating and treating persons for memory loss and dementia. A useful way of finding such qualified professionals is to contact the local chapter of the Alzheimer's Association (www.alz.org; phone: [800] 272-3900). When you contact the doctor or practitioner, ask if he or she has been trained in dementia assessment. Ask if he or she thinks it is important to check memory annually to detect Alzheimer's disease or another cause of memory loss early. If they say no or say there are not sufficient data to be sure, see someone else.

Patient History

The patient's history is a recounting of the person's problem in the overall context of his or her life. A history from the patient helps the doctor assess a person's past and current health status. It also helps the doctor evaluate whether there are any medical problems or medications contributing to the problem, develop a treatment plan, and monitor the patient's overall health over time. During this evaluation, the doctor asks the person and/or family members a series of questions. When there is concern about memory problems or dementia, it is essential to have family members present. Often the person affected is unaware of the problems and may deny or minimize them. A detailed history is essential to uncovering problems. Unfortunately, in today's managed care climate, doctors are forced to see more and more patients in less and less time, and the history often gets shortchanged. A comprehensive patient history should include

- Information about the main problem
  - What were the first symptoms to appear?
  - Did anything seem to bring it on?
  - How does it specifically interfere with your daily activities?
  - How does it specifically interfere with your more complex skills or pastimes?
  - How much is it interfering with your life?
  - Are you needing assistance from others to compensate for it?
  - When did it start?

- How rapidly did it appear?
- How rapidly has it progressed?
- How has it progressed? (gotten better, not changed, gradually declined, changed unevenly with periods of marked improvement, stabilization, or decline, periods of sudden decline with or without full recovery, and so on)
- What makes it better?
- What makes it worse?
- What other problems developed after the initial ones?
- List of all medications (many medications can cause memory problems)
- List of all vitamins, herbs, and dietary supplements (these may interact with any current medications or ones the doctor will prescribe)
- List of all current health problems
- Past medical history, including
  - Head injuries; even minor ones may be significant
  - Past surgeries or exposure to general anesthesia
  - Toxic exposures, such as work, environmental, or wartime exposure; oxygen deprivation
- Drug, alcohol, smoking history
- Sleep pattern (chronic insomnia and sleep apnea are associated with memory problems)
- Psychosocial history (marital status, living conditions, employment, sexual history, important life events)
- Family history (including any illnesses that seem to run in the family)
- Mental status exam (a series of questions and observations about appearance, speech, orientation, memory, mood, thought processes, delusions, hallucinations, social behavior, and judgment and problem solving)

Trigger Symptoms

Difficulty with any of the following activities requires assessment (we have included the area of the brain that is likely to be involved):

Learning new information: trouble remembering recent conversations, events, appointments, misplaces objects (hippocampus and entorhinal cortex)

Handling complex tasks: trouble following a complex train of thought or performing tasks that require many steps, such as balancing a checkbook or cooking a meal (prefrontal cortex)

Reasoning ability: decreased ability to respond with a reasonable plan to problems at work or home, such as knowing what to do if bathroom is flooded; poor social contact or trouble reading social cues (prefrontal cortex)

Spatial ability and orientation: trouble driving, organizing objects around the house, finding way around familiar place (parietal lobes)

Language: increased difficulty finding the words to express what he or she wants to say and with following conversations (temporal lobes and frontal lobes)

Behavior: Patient appears more passive and less responsive, is more irritable than usual, is more suspicious than usual, misinterprets visual or auditory stimuli (prefrontal and temporal lobes),

Difficulty discussing current events in an area of interest (hippocampus) or *failure to arrive* at the right time for appointments (prefrontal cortex)

Differentiating Dementia from Normal Aging

The patient history will give important clues to whether or not a serious problem is present. The following are complaints many people give with typical aging:

- Complains of memory loss but provides considerable detail regarding the events
- More concerned about the alleged memory loss than family members
- Recent memory for important events, affairs, and conversations is not impaired
- Has only occasional word-finding difficulties
- Does not get lost traveling to familiar places

- Gets lost traveling to unfamiliar places .
- Able to operate common appliances
- Maintains prior level of social skills
- Normal performance on mental status examinations

The following is a list of complaints many people and family members have when there is more serious trouble. The affected person:

- Is more dependent on others than he or she used to be
- Complains of memory problems only if specifically asked
- Is unable to recall recent conversations
- Is unable to recall recent events they attended that they enjoyed
- Is unable to recall where he or she has recently traveled to
- Frequently asks the same question several minutes later
- Is less aware of his or her memory loss than close family or friends
- Becomes more withdrawn than in the past
- Loses interest or gives up previously enjoyed activities without a good reason
- Seems to talk less
- Frequently can't find the right word for what he or she wants to say
- Gets lost traveling to familiar places
- Has greater difficulty operating appliances, remote controls, or other gadgets that he or she previously knew how to use
- Has greater difficulty learning to operate a new appliance that has replaced an old one that he or she could use well
- Starts to behave in ways that are very out of character
- Has trouble passing the written driving exam or other relatively simple tests

Depression and Attention Deficit Disorder

Depression and adult attention deficit disorder are important causes of memory problems as we age, so it is important to know how to screen for them. With depression, unlike younger adults, who may complain of a sad or depressed mood, older depressed patients may present with cognitive impairment—that is, confusion, memory disturbance, or attention deficits—all of which can be mistaken for dementia. Depression may co-exist with dementia and exacerbate the problem, increasing the disability. A thorough history and mental status examination is the first step. The *Diagnostic and Statistical Manual of Mental Disorders* (4th edition; DSM–IV) of the American Psychiatric Association requires for a diagnosis of depression that a patient experience five (or more) of the following symptoms during the same two-week period (every day for most of the day or nearly every day). At least one of the symptoms is either depressed mood or loss of interest or pleasure.

1. Depressed mood most of the time, as indicated by either subjective report (e.g., feels sad) or observation by others (e.g., appears tearful)
2. Diminished interest or pleasure in nearly all activities
3. Significant weight loss or weight gain (e.g., more than 5 percent of body weight in a month) or decrease or increase in appetite
4. Insomnia or hypersomnia
5. Psychomotor agitation or retardation
6. Fatigue or loss of energy
7. Feelings of worthlessness or guilt
8. Diminished ability to think or concentrate, or indecisiveness
9. Recurrent thoughts of death (not just fear of dying), recurrent suicidal ideation without a specific plan, or a suicide attempt or a specific plan for committing suicide

The symptoms must cause clinically significant distress or impairment in social and occupational functioning; not be due to the direct physiological effects of a substance or a general medical condition; not be better accounted for by bereavement; and persist for longer than two months or be characterized by marked functional impairment, morbid preoccupation with worthlessness, suicidal ideation, psychotic symptoms, or psychomotor retardation.

SPECT scans can usually distinguish depression from dementia. Depressed persons have increased limbic activity (deep structures in the brain) and decreased prefrontal and sometimes temporal activity at rest.

The prefrontal activity improves with concentration. The only cause of dementia that can mimic depression is frontal temporal lobe dementia. However, the scans of FTLD patients do not show increased prefrontal cortical activity with concentration.

Attention deficit disorder is characterized by short attention span, distractibility, disorganization, procrastination, and often restlessness and impulse control problems. It is often associated with learning disabilities. It used to be thought of as a childhood disorder mainly of hyperactive boys, but recently it has become clear that it affects adults. The primary problem with ADD seen on SPECT scans is decreased activity in the prefrontal cortex during concentration. It is as if the brain betrays the ADD person and shuts down when the person tries to use it. Psychostimulant medications are the most widely prescribed treatment, as they prevent the prefrontal cortex from shutting down during concentration. Over a lifetime, chronic deactivation or shutdown of the prefrontal cortex is bad for the brain and may cause atrophy or shrinkage of the brain areas involved.

The following are the DSM-IV criteria for ADD. A person must have six characteristics in either the first section, Inattentive, or the second section, Hyperactive-Impulsive, to be diagnosed as having ADD. ADD, combined type, is diagnosed by having at least six characteristics in both sections. For older adults, many of the characteristics under Hyperactive-Impulse may not be present now. However, they may have been observed during elementary school and perhaps recorded in school records.

Inattention

1. Often fails to give close attention to details or makes careless mistakes in schoolwork, work, or other activities
2. Often has difficulty sustaining attention in tasks or play activities
3. Often does not seem to listen when spoken to directly
4. Often does not follow through on instructions and fails to finish schoolwork, chores, or duties in the workplace (not due to oppositional behavior or failure to understand directions)
5. Often has difficulty organizing tasks and activities
6. Often avoids, dislikes, or is reluctant to engage in tasks that require sustained mental effort (such as schoolwork or homework)

7. Often loses things necessary for tasks or activities at school, home, or the workplace (e.g., toys, school assignments, pencils, books, or tools)
8. Often gets easily distracted by extraneous stimuli
9. Often becomes forgetful during daily activities

Hyperactivity-Impulsive (Did the teenager or adult exhibit these behaviors in elementary school?)
1. Often fidgets with hands or feet or squirms in seat
2. Often leaves seat in classroom or in other situations in which remaining seated is expected
3. Often runs about or climbs excessively in situations where it is inappropriate (in adolescents or adults, may be limited to subjective feelings of restlessness)
4. Often has difficulty playing or engaging in leisure activities quietly
5. Is often "on the go" or often acts as if "driven by motor"
6. Often talks excessively
7. Often blurts out answers before questions have been completed
8. Often has difficulty awaiting turn
9. Often interrupts or intrudes on others (e.g., butts into conversations or games)

Both depression and ADD are highly treatable illnesses. Treating them, even in the face of other dementia processes, can bring significant improvement to the lives of patients and their families.

Medication-Induced Problems

Medications can also cause serious cognitive problems. It is essential that you tell the physician every medication you take, including prescription and nonprescription ones, and have them checked to see if they may be causing problems. Bring all over-the-counter medications, herbal remedies, nutritional supplements, and prescription medications to the appointment. The following is a partial list of common medications that cause cognitive problems.

- *Antiarrhythmic Agents:* disopyramide, quinidine, tocainide
- *Antibiotics:* cephalexin, cephalothin, metronidazole, ciprofloxacin, ofloxacin
- *Anticholinergic Agents:* benztropine, homatropine, scopolamine, trihexyphenidyl
- *Anticonvulsants:* phenytoin, valproic acid, carbamazepine, Topamax
- *Antidepressants:* amitryptyline, imipramine, desipramine, trazodone, doxepin, and to a much lesser extent SSRIs, such as Prozac, Zoloft, Celexa, Paxil, and Luvox
- *Antiemetics:* promethazine, hydroxyzine, metroclopramide, prochlorperazine
- *Antihistamines/Decongestants:* phenylpropanalamine, diphenhydramine, clorpheniramine, brompheniramine, pseudoephedrine
- *Antihypertensive agents:* propranolol, metoprolol, atenolol, verapamil, methyldopa, prazosin, nifedipine; however, low doses of these medications do not typically impair cognition
- *Antimanic agents:* lithium
- *Antineoplastic agents:* chlorambucil, cytarabine, interleukin-2
- *Anti-Parkinsonian agents:* levodopa, pergolide, bromocryptine
- *Antipsychotics:* haloperidol, chlorpromazine, thioridazine
- *Cardiotonic agents:* digitalis
- *Corticosteroids:* prednisone
- *H_2 receptor antagonists:* cimetidine, ranitidine
- *Immunosuppresive agents:* cyclosporine, interferon
- *Muscle relaxants:* baclofen, cyclobenzaprine, methocarbamol
- *Narcotic analgesics:* codeine, hydrocodone, oxycodone, meperidine, propoxyphene
- *Sedatives:* alprazolam, diazepam, lorazepam, flurazepam, clonazepam, phenobarbital, chloral hydrate

Physical Exam

A physical examination is an important part of the evaluation process. The exam enables the doctor to assess the overall physical condition of the patient. If the patient has a medical complaint, the physical exam provides the doctor with more information about the problem, which helps him determine an appropriate plan of treatment. The physical exam includes an examination of the following:

- General observations—appearance, skin color
- Vital signs (temperature, blood pressure, and pulse lying and standing)
- Height and weight
- Skin
- Head, eyes, ears, nose
- Throat/neck
- Chest, including lungs and heart
- Breasts
- Abdomen
- Bones and muscles
- Nerves/reflexes
- Rectal/genital area

Laboratory tests

When physicians are concerned about a problem, they often order laboratory tests on certain fluids and tissue samples from the body. These tests can help identify problems and diseases. There are hundreds of laboratory tests available to help doctors make a diagnosis. The most common are blood tests and urinalysis. Blood tests involve a series of tests that are routinely done on blood to look for abnormalities associated with various diseases and disorders.

Blood tests may also be used to look for the presence of a specific gene that has been linked to Alzheimer's disease. A urinalysis is a test in which a urine sample is evaluated to detect abnormalities, such as abnormal levels of sugar or protein. This test may be used by the doctor to help rule out other disorders that may be causing symptoms similar to those of Alzheimer's disease.

Common laboratory tests:

- Urinalysis—to look for kidney disease that can contribute to dementia
- Complete blood count (CBC)—to look for low blood count or anemia diseases

- Liver function tests (AST, ALT, alkaline phosphatase, bilirubin)
- Folate levels—for folic acid deficiencies that affect nerve cell function
- Homocysteine level—elevated level is a risk factor for strokes and Alzheimer's disease; folic acid supplementation helps to bring the level down
- Vitamin B_{12} level—to look for B_{12} deficiency from small intestine absorption problems
- Electrolyte and blood glucose levels (sodium, potassium, creatinine, glucose, calcium)—to look for metabolic problems, kidney, liver, gallbladder, bone, glandular, and blood vessel diseases
- Thyroid function tests; abnormal thyroid hormone levels are a common cause of forgetfulness, confusion, lethargy, and other symptoms of dementia in older women and men; medication can easily improve symptoms if a thyroid problem is present
- Syphilis screening; dementia is a symptom of late-stage syphilis; if the person had syphilis many years ago and was never properly treated, the illness may have progressed to the point of affecting behavior and intelligence; although syphilis is uncommon, this test is often used when there is a history of multiple sexual contacts.
- Test for human immunodeficiency virus (HIV) infection, if the person has multiple sexual partners or is from sub-Saharan Africa
- Erythrocyte sedimentation rate—to look for inflammatory, infectious, autoimmune, or blood diseases
- Apolipoprotein E genotype—to check genetic risk; the presence of the ApoE4 gene, as discussed previously, significantly increases a person's risk for Alzheimer's disease and makes symptoms appear five to ten years earlier than in the general population. Many children of an affected parent wish to know the parent's apolipoprotein E genotype so they can determine their chance of inheriting a higher risk for AD, atherosclerosis, heart disease, and stroke.
- Fasting lipid panel—high total cholesterol and LDL is a risk factor
- For a man, it may be worthwhile getting a testosterone level test, particularly if over age 75 or if there are symptoms of fatigue, weakness, docile behavior, or reduced libido.

- For a woman after menopause, it may be worthwhile getting an estradiol level (a form of estrogen), particularly if she does not take estrogen replacement therapy.
- If sleep problems are present and a clear cause is not established, then a sleep study in a designated sleep lab may be important. Sleep apnea has been reported to cause serious problems in the parietal lobes of the brain, one of the areas affected in Alzheimer's disease.

Electrocardiogram (ECG or EKG)

An electrocardiogram is a recording of the heart's electrical activity. This activity is registered as a graph or series of wavy lines on a moving strip of paper. This gives the doctor important information about the heart. For example, it can show the heart's rate and rhythm. It also can help show decreased blood flow, enlargement of the heart, or the presence of damage due to a current or past heart attack. This test may be used by the doctor to help rule out other conditions that may be causing symptoms similar to those of Alzheimer's disease.

Chest X-Ray

X-rays can be used to diagnose a wide range of conditions, from bronchitis to broken bones. When viewing X-ray images of the chest, doctors can view the structures inside the chest, including the heart, lungs, and bones. This test may be used by the doctor to help rule out other disorders that may be causing symptoms similar to those of Alzheimer's disease.

Imaging Brain Activity: Single Photon Emission Computed Tomography (SPECT) and Positron Emission Tomography (PET)

As we have discussed, SPECT is a technique for creating very clear, three-dimensional pictures of the brain; SPECT scans show how the brain functions, unlike X-ray, CT, or MRI images, which show only body structure. The SPECT scan involves the injection of a very small amount of a radioactive substance into the bloodstream, and energy from the radioactive substance in the body is detected by a special camera, which then takes the pictures. This procedure can be used to see how blood flows in certain regions of the brain and is useful in evaluating specific brain functions. A SPECT scan may reveal abnormalities that are characteristic of Alzheimer's disease or other forms of memory problems.

Recent studies suggest that SPECT can identify persons with reduced brain activity years before they actually lose brain tissue. The reduced brain activity correlates very well with objective impairment on cognitive testing, both of which can identify early-stage ADRD up to four years before the first symptoms appear. After the history, physical exam, and blood work are done, an MRI of the brain should be done to identify hydrocephalus, tumors, vascular causes of dementia, or selective hippocampal tissue loss in AD and to identify other patterns of tissue loss characteristic of FTLD and LBD.

If the diagnosis remains uncertain or one wants to assess the degree of abnormal brain activity prior to treatment, then an image of the brain's activity should be done using SPECT or PET scanning. A principal advantage of SPECT over PET scanning in ADRD evaluation is that SPECT is reimbursed by Medicare and many other insurers, while PET is not.

A PET scan is quite similar to SPECT. The primary differences between them are that they use different radioactive molecules to measure brain activity and that PET scanners detect positrons emitting from these radioactive molecules, whereas SPECT scanners detect emitting photons. The precision of a PET scan is better than a SPECT scan, but not enough to make a clinical difference in ADRD diagnosis, disease monitoring, and monitoring of treatment efficacy. A resting SPECT scan typically costs under $1,000, and a resting PET scan typically costs $1,200 to $2,000. With newer cameras, SPECT scanning time is under 15 minutes, while PET scanning time is 30 minutes.

Magnetic Resonance Imaging (MRI)

This is a scan that uses a large magnet, radio waves, and a computer to produce pictures of the structure of the brain without using X-rays. Structural changes in the brain seen in ADRD include tissue loss (atrophy), tumors, swelling of the ventricles (hydrocephalus), strokes and loss of the myelin wrapping around neurons (demyelination). An MRI of the brain is about a thousand times more sensitive than a CT scan. A structural image of the brain is essential in diagnosing ADRD. A normal MRI of the brain means that the underlying cause of cognitive impairment has not progressed to the point where brain tissue has died. In this case, SPECT or PET are the best methods of detecting abnormal changes in brain activity that will allow the earliest diagnosis to be accurately made and allow the most effective ADRD treatments to be given.

Neuropsychological Testing

Neuropsychological testing measures the function of brain areas that interpret one's environment, make decisions, and decide how to act on them. The following is a partial listing of the kinds of abilities that neuropsychologic tests measure:

Neuropsychologic tests of vision: color perception, line orientation, tracking the motion of objects, object recognition, face recognition

Neuropsychologic tests of hearing: tone perception, pitch discrimination, word recognition, comprehension, naming presented objects, fluency of speech, fluency of ability to generate words belonging to specific categories

Neuropsychologic tests of memory: immediate recall, recall after several minutes delay, recall of events from the past, recalling the names of familiar objects, recalling the names of well-known concepts

Neuropsychologic tests of the frontal lobes: attention, shifting between tasks, judgment, reasoning, estimation, ability to execute complex sequences of movements

While he was clinical director of the University of California, Irvine, Alzheimer's Disease Research Center, Dr. Shankle, along with Dr. Dick, the center's chief neuropsychologist, reviewed the test results of over four hundred patients who had received a SPECT scan. On the basis of the neuropsychologic test results, Dr. Dick would draw a picture of where the impairments were in the brain. They would then compare this picture with the SPECT brain activity images. What was remarkable was that the areas of reduced brain activity on the SPECT scans were almost always identical to the areas identified by Dr. Dick's analysis of the neuropsychologic test results.

The two methods, SPECT and neuropsychologic testing, are highly complementary and provide a reliable measure of the state of an individual's brain function. Both can detect abnormalities in brain function up to four years before you are able to notice the first difficulty in performing a specific ability. In this sense, they are invaluable early detection tools that can be used to confirm a positive screening test result. They can be used as part of the standard workup or can be used if the standard workup does not identify the underlying problem. The combination of SPECT scanning and neuropsychologic testing can also provide families with a much better understanding of the reasons that their loved one is behaving the way he or she does. For example, instead of accusing the person of denial or not wanting to remember something, they understand that the damage in the hippocampus prevents the person from recording the event so that it literally never happened. The short-term memory testing confirmed that the person recalled none of the information he or she learned even just a few minutes later.

Establishing the correct diagnosis, while it may be costly, is money well spent. Without it, families can spend thousands of dollars on the wrong treatment while the person's disease progresses. The earlier and better informed you are, the better able you will be to take proper action and seek effective treatment.

Treatment for Mild Memory Loss and Early Alzheimer's and Related Disorders

❁ Recently, a subcommittee of the American Academy of Neurology reviewed the published data on the costs and benefits of detecting dementia early. On the basis of this review, they recommended that people with mild cognitive impairment be further evaluated, monitored, and if progressing, diagnosed and treated. Mild cognitive impairment is now known to greatly increase the risk of developing dementia.

Current methods of prevention and treatment can significantly delay both the onset of symptoms and the progression of ADRD. Through a combination of family education, drug therapy, antioxidant therapy, and lifestyle changes, the effects of AD, as well as many of the other ADRD causes of dementia, can be significantly delayed. The result is improved quality of life and reduced costs and burden on loved ones for assisted care.

Table 8.1. Impairment Levels for CDRS Scores			
	None (0)	**Questionable (0.5)**	
Memory	No memory loss or slight inconsistent forgetfulness	Consistent slight forgetfulness; partial recollection of events	
Orientation	Fully oriented	Fully oriented, except for slight difficulty with time relationships	
Judgment and problem solving	Solves everyday problems and handles business and financial affairs well; judgment good in relation to past performance	Slight impairment in solving problems, similarities, and differences	
Community affairs	Independent function at usual level in job, shopping, volunteer and social groups	Slight impairment in these activities	
Home and hobbies	Life at home, hobbies, and intellectual interests well maintained	Life at home, hobbies, and intellectual interests slightly impaired	
Personal care	Fully capable of self-care		

According to Dr. Howard M. Fillit, the executive director of the Institute for the Study of Aging, "in the long term, drug therapy for AD reduces overall expenses by decreasing hospitalization and institutionalization rates, diminishing caregiver burden, and helping to control costly and debilitating complications of AD" (27). Studies on AD treatment show that a greater degree of cognitive impairment at the time of diagnosis is associated with higher total cost of care and longer stays in a nursing home.

Unfortunately, almost all cases of mild ADRD go undetected until the patient is moderately demented. The research of Dr. Jeffrey Cummings, director of the Alzheimer's disease program at the University of California, Los Angeles, found that more than 95 percent of people in the mild stages

Mild (1)	Moderate (2)	Severe (3)
Moderate memory loss; more marked for recent events; defect interferes with everyday activities	Severe memory loss; only highly learned material retained; new material rapidly lost	Severe memory loss; only fragments remain
Moderate difficulty with time relationships; oriented for place at examination; may have geographic disorientation elsewhere	Severe difficulty with time relationships; usually disoriented to time, often to place	Oriented to person only
Moderate difficulty in handling problems, similarities, and differences; social judgment usually maintained	Severely impaired in handling problems, similarities, and differences; social judgment usually impaired	Unable to make judgments or solve problems
Unable to function independently at these activities, although may still be engaged in some; appears normal to casual inspection	No pretense of independent function outside home Appears well enough to be taken to functions outside a family home	No pretense of independent function outside home Appears too ill to be taken to functions outside a family home
Mild but definite impairment of function at home; more difficult chores abandoned; more complicated hobbies and interests abandoned	Only simple chores preserved; very restricted interests, poorly maintained	No significant function in home
Needs prompting	Requires assistance in dressing, hygiene, keeping of personal effects	Requires much help with personal care; frequent incontinence

of dementia are not detected in primary care physician practices (76). Symptoms are usually present for four years before dementia is detected, by which time it is in the moderate stages and is halfway through the average eight-year course of AD. Slowing ADRD progression in a moderately demented person is much less satisfactory, which is probably why AD is treated for an average of only six months; AD treatment is stopped, in spite of the fact that medical research shows it to be effective in delaying disease progression even into the severe stages.

The terms *mild cognitive impairment, mild dementia,* and *moderate dementia* are misleading because they have a specific meaning to medical researchers and a totally different meaning to others. Researchers measure dementia severity with a standardized scale, the most common of which is the Clinical Dementia Rating Scale (CDRS). The CDRS categorizes dementia severity into one of six classes:

- 0: normal
- 0.5: very mild or questionable dementia (sometimes also called mild cognitive impairment)
- 1: mild dementia
- 2: moderate dementia
- 3: severe dementia
- 4: terminal dementia

Treating Early Disease: General Recommendations

There are treatment recommendations that apply to all causes of dementia due to ADRD that can delay their progression, keep people independent, and reduce the burden on their families. We use these general recommendations for all our cognitively impaired or demented patients.

Exercise

Because of the effects of exercise on many different factors that determine ADRD progression, people who regularly exercise almost always maintain their abilities longer than people who do not. There is simply no good reason not to find some form of exercise that can be done for 20 to 30 minutes each day to both prevent cognitive decline with aging, and to delay decline if cognitive impairment or dementia already exists.

Antioxidants

Free radicals damage nerve cells as well as trigger self-destruct genes to kill neurons in virtually every brain disease of aging. As antioxidants decline with age, people with mild ADRD are even more vulnerable to disease progression through neuron damage and death by free radicals. This is why we treat every ADRD patient with antioxidants at doses that are often much higher than those indicated for normal aging people. There are some differences in the specific antioxidants used for the different causes of dementia due to ADRD; these specific differences will be mentioned in the treatment sections for each ADRD cause. However, for all the causes of ADRD discussed in this chapter, the following antioxidants may help slow disease progression.

Alpha Lipoic Acid (ALA): 300 to 600 mg twice a day

In studies measuring the ability of ALA to repair nerve damage in diabetics, 100 mg a day was ineffective. Doses of 600 and 1,200 mg a day were effective and well tolerated, but the 1,200 mg dose had slightly more side effects. There is only one small study of ALA in AD people, which suggested that it delayed disease progression. However, because ALA is the most effective antioxidant in raising glutathione levels in the cell (which is the cell's major line of defense against damage by free radicals) and because it is well tolerated, it may be the best antioxidant for people with ADRD.

Vitamin C: 250-500 mg twice a day, taken with vitamin E (mixed tocopherols; dose depends on the cause of the ADRD)

Vitamin C recycles vitamin E to make it more effective as an antioxidant and protect vulnerable brain areas from damage by AD. Vitamin E (alpha tocopherol) in doses of 1,000 i.u. twice a day was studied in a large multicenter trial of AD patients. After carefully adjusting for factors that might obscure its effect, they found that vitamin E at this dose delayed AD progression by almost one year. The mixed tocopherol preparations of vitamin E (which are also found in fruits and vegetables) are more effective antioxidants than the alpha tocopherol form of vitamin E (the type most commonly sold in stores). Given the choice, it is probably better to take the mixed tocopherol form of vitamin E, either as a supplement or through your diet.

Nicotine

Animal models of AD, as well as aging, have shown that nicotine increases neurotransmitter release. In neurons, nicotine increases glutamate release, which increases electrical activity of the receiving neuron to make learning and memory easier. Since short-term memory is usually a big problem early on in all ADRD diseases, nicotine can be very helpful. Nicotine can be given as chewing gum, a nasal spray, or a skin patch. Also, Reminyl, one of the treatments for AD, activates nicotine receptors and can be used to improve working or short-term memory.

When very mild dementia or mild cognitive impairment is treated with nicotine, it can significantly improve working or short-term memory. Dr. Shankle has treated many such people with a nicotine patch (7 mg put on in the morning and taken off at bedtime for two weeks, then increasing to 14 mg a day for two weeks if no ill effect and well tolerated, then increasing to 21 mg a day for two weeks if no ill effect and well tolerated, then stopping if no ill effect). The nicotine chewing gum can also be used, but many people do not like the taste. Another way to deliver nicotine to the brain is to take Reminyl. When Reminyl is the treatment of choice for the particular individual, then nicotine patches are not needed. Dr. Shankle has often effectively used nicotine patches in very mildly impaired people when the treatment of choice is Exelon. In some people who give up a favorite activity that depends on working or short-term memory, such as reading, treatment with nicotine can restore the activity. One patient who had AD for eight years suddenly gave up reading. After starting her on nicotine, she resumed reading within two weeks and continued to enjoy it for another two years.

Memantine (Namenda)

Memantine is produced by Merz Pharmaceuticals in Germany and has been used in Europe since the 1990s as one of the approved treatments for AD. In 2003, Forest Laboratories obtained the rights to distribute Memantine under the name Namenda in the United States. Since it will be known as Namenda in the United States, we will use that term. The Food and Drug Administration has approved Namenda for use in moderate to severe AD. It became available in January 2004. Namenda may be useful in improving function for a variety of causes of dementia due to ADRD. It has recently been shown to improve symptoms as well as to delay the progression of moderate to severe AD.

Namenda partly blocks the N-methyl D-aspartate (NMDA) receptor to reduce the entry of too much calcium into neurons, which protects them from damage. Calcium is the critical factor in controlling the activity of virtually every cell in your body, which is why calcium is strongly regulated inside cells. In fact, calcium is one billion times more concentrated inside cells than outside them! When activated by learning new information or learning a new skill, the NMDA receptor binds the neurotransmitter glutamate and increases the entry of calcium and sodium into the receiving neuron. This increased entry of calcium and sodium increases the voltage of the receiving neuron to make it more likely that it will pass the message onto the next neuron, so that you are more likely to learn the new information or skill. However, a large number of brain diseases cause too much glutamate to be released, which causes too much calcium to enter neurons, which triggers a cascade of excessive enzyme activity that ultimately turns on genes that are programmed to kill the neuron. This doesn't mean you should stop taking calcium or drinking milk or having other dairy products. Under normal circumstances, your cells can handle the calcium in foods without triggering programmed cell death.

With this in mind, Namenda may block the programmed cell death that occurs in the various diseases that trigger excessive release of the neurotransmitter glutamate. This means that Namenda may slow the progression of AD, stroke and vascular dementia, epilepsy, frontal temporal lobe dementia, and presumably others. However, at present, the evidence that Namenda blocks programmed cell death is still at the animal model level.

Clinical Experience with Namenda

Namenda can sometimes produce dramatic benefits in people with ADRD. One of the more dramatic effects of Namenda is that it reduces the spasticity that occurs in most types of ADRD as they progress: people who are rigid, off balance, and have difficulty walking or falling are able to move better. Another effect of Namenda is that it can reduce urinary incontinence. Namenda can also help improve speech and fine motor skills involved in self-care, hobbies, and household activities. When Namenda is helpful, it is quite noticeable to the family and can significantly reduce

Figures 8.1-4. Ralph's SPECT Scan, Before and After Treatment with Namenda

Underside surface views

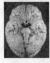
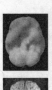
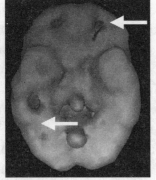
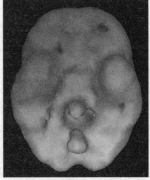

Before treatment
Decreased activity in PFC
right temporal lobe

After treatment
Overall improved activity

Underside active views

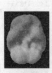
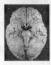
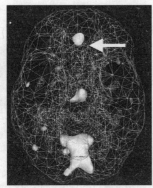
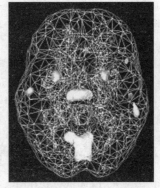
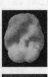
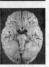

Before treatment
Increased anterior cingulate
activity (arrow)
(gets stuck on negative thoughts
or behaviors)

After treatment
Calming of anterior cingulate

their stress and the caregiving time required. Namenda is usually started with half of a 10 mg tablet in the morning for two weeks and then increased slowly to as high as 40 mg in some people.

One patient of Dr. Shankle's, Ralph, was a young man who had had a viral infection in the brain as a child. The infection left him with permanent loss of ability to perform coordinated movements, speak clearly, and behave appropriately at work or in social circumstances. He had been fired from many jobs because of this "attitude" problem. Despite being intelligent, he also had problems with learning and memory. His SPECT scan was remarkable in that the cerebellum showed almost no activity. It also showed poor activity in his prefrontal cortex (judgment, impulse control, and concentration center) and right temporal lobe (reading social cues) and increased activity in the anterior cingulate gyrus (often associated with trouble shifting attention, cognitive inflexibility, and oppositional and difficult behavior). After he had taken Namenda for three months, the family reported that he was more coordinated, spoke more clearly, and behaved more appropriately. He was able to get occupational therapy and start working again.

Another patient, Edith, was incontinent, could no longer walk, and could no longer talk. After a three-month trial of Namenda, she regained continence, was able to walk slowly on her own, and was able to communicate with her family again.

Treating Mild Cognitive Impairment or Dementia Due to Alzheimer's Disease

When Dr. Shankle began working with ADRD patients in 1988, there were no treatments available. Now we have the potential to effectively eliminate institutionalization in most people who are affected by AD if it is detected and treated early. There is extensive medical research to support our understanding of how to accomplish the disease-delaying effects of AD treatment. The following approach is based on an understanding of the current mechanisms by which AD progresses and how they can be stopped or delayed. The mainstay of AD treatment is the combination of a cholinesterase inhibitor (Exelon, Reminyl, or Aricept) with antioxidants (vitamins C and E and alpha lipoic acid).

Cholinesterase Inhibitors (Exelon, Reminyl, and Aricept)

There are important differences among the cholinesterase inhibitors that may very well determine how effectively AD can be delayed. However, their common link is that they keep an enzyme called acetylcholinesterase (AChE) from breaking down the neurotransmitter acetylcholine. This increases the amount of activity between neurons that release acetylcholine and those that receive it. Because acetylcholine neurons are found throughout the cerebral cortex of the brain, increasing acetylcholine can affect many abilities, which is exactly what the medical research has found. These medications improve activities of daily life, reduce behavioral problems, and in the mild stages of AD, improve mental abilities such as attention, short-term memory, comprehension, communication, and ability to recognize people and objects.

The specific abilities improved in each person with AD vary according to how much each ability is affected; severely impaired abilities often do not improve, which is why treating early is so important, as well as why short-term memory often does not improve in people with AD when they are first diagnosed and treated—two to four years after symptoms first begin. We have treated many AD patients who had symptoms for less than six months, and in these patients short-term memory often improves.

While improving function and reducing problems is what people most want when they see a doctor, this is only half the treatment. The other, and probably more important, half of the treatment involves delaying or halting the progression of the disease process of AD itself. It is here where Exelon, Reminyl, and Aricept differ the most.

Exelon (Rivastigmine)

While Exelon, Reminyl, and Aricept all block AChE, only Exelon blocks butyrylcholinesterase (BuChE), the other enzyme that breaks down acetyl- choline (77). In normal aging people, about 80 percent of the cholinesterase is AChE and 20 percent is BuChE. However, as AD progresses, the amount of AChE decreases and the amount of BuChE increases so that they are about equal. The reason this is important is that it appears that BuChE is the enzyme that converts amyloid precursor protein (APP) into BA42 in- side plaques to convert them into the neuritic plaques of AD. To maxi- mally block the progression of the AD disease process itself, both AChE and BuChE must be blocked. At present, the only medication that does this is Exelon, which is why it is our first choice in treating AD.

Reminyl (Galantamine)

Our second choice is Reminyl. Reminyl does not block BuChE, which means that it cannot slow the accumulation of the neuritic plaques the way Exelon can. However, Reminyl binds to nicotine receptors, which increases the levels of many different neurotransmitters to generally increase brain ac- tivity (78). Another effect of the nicotine receptor is that it may help block programmed cell death. However, this effect has only been shown in animal models, so it is not certain whether Reminyl actually blocks programmed cell death in AD or other brain diseases. If Reminyl does block pro- grammed cell death in AD, then it would slow AD progression in a way that is different from Exelon. It would then be possible to use a combina- tion of these medications to slow AD progression more effectively than ei- ther Exelon or Reminyl alone. At present, Reminyl remains a second choice because it has not been proven to block programmed cell death in AD. We have discussed this issue with the manufacturers of Reminyl, and it is hoped that they will address this important research issue.

Aricept (Donepezil)

Our third choice in treating AD is Aricept, which, ironically, is the most commonly prescribed of the three cholinesterase inhibitors, for several reasons. First, Aricept was the first well-tolerated cholinesterase inhibitor produced in the United States. Cognex (tacrine) was the first cholinesterase inhibitor approved by the Food and Drug Administration, but it had many intolerable side effects. Second, Aricept has fewer side effects than either Exelon or Reminyl. Third, Aricept only needs to be given once a day, as opposed to twice a day for Exelon and Reminyl. (In 2004, Reminyl will be available as a once-a-day formulation.) And Aricept blocks AChE, which in animal models reduces BA42 production to reduce the number of AD neuritic plaques formed. This AChE blockade is most useful in very mild to mild AD, when only about 20 percent of ChE is BuChE, and 80 percent is AChE. These advantages are attractive, particularly to busy primary care physicians. However, there are some important reasons why it is not the first choice in treating moderate to severe AD.

Aricept (like Reminyl) does not block BuChE, which is about 50 percent of the total ChE amount by the time a person is moderately demented with AD. Aricept is therefore most effective in blocking the accumulation of the neuritic plaques of AD, which is directly related to AD disease progression.

Aricept (like Exelon) does not bind to the nicotine receptor, so it does not increase overall brain activity as effectively as Reminyl and does not potentially block programmed cell death.

While many researchers remain unconvinced that blocking both BuChE and AchE is practically important in AD, Dr. Shankle has switched hundreds of moderate to severe AD patients who were declining on Aricept to Exelon. About half of these patients stopped declining and recovered some of their lost ground. This type of study is called a crossover study because individuals become their own control. It has the advantage of controlling for many factors that vary when comparing the effect of two treatments (such as drug versus placebo) on different subjects. Published research has also recently appeared that supports Dr. Shankle's findings. Approximately three hundred mildly to moderately demented AD patients who showed no benefit from Aricept were switched to Exelon and treated for six months. Of this group, half showed improvements in daily activities, behavior, and/or mental abilities on Exelon.

In summary, when people with moderate to severe AD do not tolerate Exelon and Reminyl, we put them on Aricept because it still can delay AD progression, albeit not as effectively as Exelon. Whether Aricept and Reminyl delay AD progression equally well is not known because the effect of Reminyl on blocking programmed cell death is still at the animal research level of evidence.

In very mild to mild AD, it is not yet clear whether Exelon is more effective in delaying AD progression than Aricept or Reminyl. In these milder stages, the agent that gives the best improvement in symptoms would be a reasonable choice.

Side Effects of the Cholinesterase Inhibitors

The clinical trial research on Exelon and Reminyl indicates that they have a similar frequency of side effects, which is about 11 percent. However, people who participate in clinical trials are often healthier than people who are treated in community physician practices. Dr. Shankle has seen about a 15 percent to 20 percent incidence of side effects with Exelon and Reminyl. The reported frequency of side effects with Aricept in clinical trials is generally lower, at about 5 percent.

One behavioral side effect of the cholinesterase inhibitors is that they can produce aggression, and it often occurs with improvement in mental abilities. The psychosocial explanation of aggression with improved cognition is that the improved mental abilities lead to greater awareness about one's difficulties, which leads to frustration and aggression. The neurological explanation is that a balance of norepinephrine, serotonin, acetylcholine, GABA, dopamine, opiate, and testosterone controls aggressive behavior. In AD, this complex balance can be dramatically altered, such that treating AD by increasing acetylcholine can precipitate aggression. However, when aggression occurs, families often do not want to stop or reduce the medication because their loved one is functioning so much better. In this situation, we may give an anticonvulsant or an antidepressant to combat it. Aggression usually resolves within two weeks.

The primary side effects of Exelon and Reminyl are nausea, vomiting, loss of appetite, dizziness, lightheadedness or fainting, generalized weakness, and muscle pain. While these side effects sound as though they are largely related to the stomach or heart, they are in fact related to the effect of increasing acetylcholine activity in the brain stem. In the brain stem are groups of neurons that control vomiting (to keep you from swallowing things that will kill you), breathing, heart rate, blood pressure, and metabolism. The effect of acetylcholine on the heart is to slow the heart rate, which causes a drop in blood pressure, which in turn can result in fainting, lightheadedness, or dizziness that can be severe enough to require a trip to the emergency room. It is usually not life-threatening and is managed by reducing the dose of Exelon or Reminyl to a level low enough for these symptoms not to return.

The side effects of Aricept are similar to Exelon and Reminyl but less frequent. One side effect that is unique to Aricept is the occurrence of nightmares in people who take it at bedtime. Taking it in the morning usually resolves this side effect.

Treating Mild Cognitive Impairment or Dementia Due to Vascular Disease

The primary treatment of mild forms of vascular dementia (VD) is to stop further brain damage from stroke or reduced blood flow. There are three components to treating mild VD to keep it from progressing, as follows.

1. *Thin the blood to reduce stroke risk from clotting.* Aspirin is used for this; the suggested dose is 81 mg once a day. Baby aspirin reduces the chance of future strokes by making platelets less likely to form a clot and block blood flow. When there is evidence that brain damage from reduced blood flow or strokes is continuing while taking aspirin, then adding dipyridamole (Persantine) can help. Aggrenox is a more convenient, and possibly more effective, combination of aspirin and dipyridamole and appears to be the most effective protection against stroke because it not only thins the blood but also improves blood flow to the heart to make it pump more efficiently. Aggrenox is built up to one capsule twice a day over two weeks to avoid side effects related to headache and flushing from dilated blood vessels.

For people who cannot tolerate aspirin, then Plavix, 75 mg once a day, will reduce risk of further strokes. Finally, if all these measures fail, then treatment with Coumadin, the most powerful blood thinner, may block stroke progression. Coumadin is routinely used when (1) there is severe narrowing of major blood vessels to the brain that cannot be surgically corrected; (2) there are multiple TIAs, or ministrokes, that resolve within 24 hours; or (3) there is atrial fibrillation or some other irregular heart rhythm that is likely to cause blood clots to form in the heart and cause strokes.

2. Treat the underlying risk factors for VD. See Chapter 3, page 48, for a discussion of the specific risk factors for VD. Each risk factor you have that contributes to stroke risk should be treated as effectively as possible.

3. Increase blood flow from the heart to the brain. The factors that determine how much blood flows out of the heart are the strength of heart muscle contraction when it ejects blood; the volume of blood in the heart when it contracts; the percentage of blood inside the heart that actually leaves the heart when it contracts; and the number of times per minute the heart beats.

Exercise is by far the most important treatment that will improve the heart's ability to pump blood to the brain. Other correctable factors that can improve heart output are:

- Minimizing the amount of blood regurgitated back into the heart because of damaged heart valves
- Reducing the resistance to blood ejected from the heart by controlling blood pressure
- Treating irregular rhythms to improve blood filling and leaving the heart
- Treating anemia to prevent reduced blood delivery to the heart and elsewhere

Treating Symptoms

Cholinesterase Inhibitors (Exelon, Reminyl, and Aricept)

Of the three cholinesterase inhibitors, Aricept and Reminyl have completed clinical trials of people with mild to moderate VD. Both Aricept and Reminyl improve some of the symptoms of VD. An interesting finding from these studies is that people with AD who also have vascular disease in the brain, which is the case about one-third of the time, respond better to treatment than people with AD without vascular disease.

Based on Reminyl's ability to activate nicotine receptors and increase overall brain activity, our first choice in treating VD is Reminyl. If Reminyl is ineffective, then either Aricept or Exelon should be tried. Since Reminyl is basically Aricept plus the additional effect of nicotine receptor modulation, it may be that Exelon would be a better second choice. However, there are no data presently to show whether this is the case.

A side benefit of the cholinesterase inhibitors in treating VD is that they appear to increase blood flow to the brain in animal models.

See page 191 for side effects of these medications.

Attention Deficit Disorder Drugs

Because VD impairs the frontal lobes more than other areas of the brain, difficulty concentrating, paying attention, planning, organizing, or completing tasks is often significantly affected. These difficulties are heavily dependent on working memory and resemble those seen in children and adults with attention deficit disorder. Working memory problems often respond to medications that increase dopamine and norepinephrine activity in the frontal lobes. Such medications include the psychostimulants Adderall, Dexedrine, Concerta, Focalin, Ritalin, and Strattera (a new agent that is almost a pure norepinephrine agent).

For people with heart disease, the safest of these agents is Focalin. For people without heart disease and with fatigue or very low energy, Adderall tends to be more effective. Other individuals without heart disease and without significant loss of energy or fatigue should be tried on regular Ritalin first to find the optimal dose. Once the optimal dose is found, a trial of a sustained-release form of Ritalin, such as Ritalin LA or Concerta, can be done to compare whether sustained release or regular release is more effective. Sometimes people use a sustained-release form in the morning and add a regular release dose in the afternoon to get a more even response during the day.

Because the treatment for short-term memory loss is different (i.e., to give a cholinesterase inhibitor with or without nicotine) from that for working memory, it is important to distinguish between them so the right treatment can be given. Henry is a good example of the benefits of treating the right kind of memory impairment as well as the benefits of exercise in VD.

Henry ❖

At 79, Henry had a mild case of VD. Because he was 79 years old and had a number of risk factors that would reduce blood flow to his brain, Dr. Shankle recommended that Henry gradually increase the time on his Exercycle from his usual 10 minutes a day to a minimum of 30 minutes every day. Over the next few months, he increased his exercise to 40 minutes a day. During this time, he noted gradual improvement in executing real estate transactions.

Unfortunately, his working memory span was still affected, and he had difficulty retrieving names. Therefore, he was given a small dose of Focalin, a form of methylphenidate that is relatively safer for the heart. Almost immediately he showed improvement in name retrieval and a marked ability to concentrate. The observation was confirmed with objective follow-up testing of his cognition and brain activity with SPECT scanning.

Figures 8.5-6. Before and After Treatment with Stimulants (Adderall)

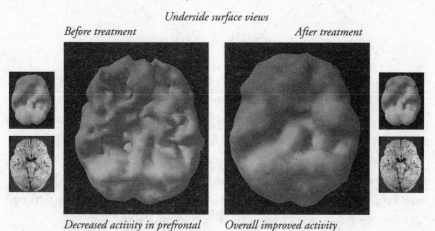

Underside surface views

Before treatment   *After treatment*

Decreased activity in prefrontal cortex right temporal lobe   *Overall improved activity*

Treating Mild Lewy Body Disease

Like VD, Lewy body disease (LBD) coexists with AD somewhere between 10 percent and 30 percent of the time. (For a complete description of LBD, see Chapter 3, page 39.) People with mild LBD frequently experience one or more of the following symptoms:

- Marked fluctuations, over hours to days, in focus, organization attention, mental clarity, or alertness
- Difficulty with balance, putting one foot in front of the other, or coordinated movement
- Marked slowing of responses to others during conversation
- Marked visual changes or hallucinations
- Marked change in rapid eye movement (REM) stage sleep and possibly vivid dreams or nightmares

The reason for this pattern of symptoms early in LBD is that it affects the occipital lobes, which process simple visual features such as lines, colors, and depth; the frontal lobes, which control attention, concentration, and speed and coordination of movement; and the substantia nigra in the midbrain of the brain stem, which affects movement and level of consciousness (mental alertness) and is the primary area of damage in Parkinson's disease.

Coenzyme Q10

At present, there is no known treatment to slow the accumulation of the Lewy bodies associated with LBD (the deposit of the substances is thought to be a significant part of the cause of LBD). However, it has recently been shown that CoQ10 substantially delays the progression of Parkinson's disease when given early. Because Parkinson's disease and LBD both share the accumulation of Lewy bodies in the brain, treatment with CoQ10 may also help slow the progression of LBD. At present, no specific clinical trials have been done to examine the effect of CoQ10 in LBD.

Cholinesterase Inhibitors

The symptoms of LBD can respond dramatically to treatment with cholinesterase inhibitors. Aricept, Reminyl, and Exelon have all been shown to improve hallucinations, attention, daytime drowsiness, disturbed sleep, walking, and other motor coordination problems associated with LBD. To date, the most extensive clinical studies of treatment response in LBD have been done with Exelon. The longest study showed that Exelon initially produced dramatic improvement in behavioral and mental function and, over the course of the two-year study, prevented people with LBD from declining below their pretreatment baseline condition. This finding suggests that Exelon, at least, may keep people with LBD from declining for two or more years.

Aricept has been examined in only a handful of LBD patients and has shown benefits. However, because people with LBD have the largest reduction of acetylcholine in their brains, Exelon and Reminyl have the theoretical advantage of being able to produce greater increases in acetylcholine. This may explain why only about half of the 13 reported people with LBD treated with Aricept responded to treatment. To date, there are no studies of Reminyl in treating LBD, although one is in progress. However, it should be more effective than Aricept. At present, until more information comparing Exelon and Reminyl in treating LBD is available and LBD disease mechanisms are better defined, our treatment preferences for LBD are Exelon as first treatment choice, Reminyl second, and Aricept third.

Treating Psychosis in LBD

Psychosis refers to the presence of hallucinations, illusions, or delusions. *Visual hallucinations* means seeing things that are not there, and this is very common in LBD. *Illusions* are misinterpretations of what one sees—for example, mistaking a shadow in the house for a stranger. *Delusions* are irrational ideas that a person cannot be convinced are false (e.g., that the person's dead parents are living in the house). Visual hallucinations and delusions in LBD are related to reduced acetylcholine transmission in areas of the temporal lobe that recognize objects and figures, as well as increased numbers of dopamine receptors on basal ganglia neurons that receive dopamine input from the brain stem (substantia nigra). These changes suggest several treatment strategies for psychosis in LBD.

Exelon or Aricept increase the level of acetylcholine by blocking its breakdown. Exelon works particularly well when side effects do not occur. Aricept is likely to be effective when the numbers of acetylcholine receptors are not severely reduced, as would occur in early-stage LBD.

Reminyl and nicotine increase nicotine activation and acetylcholine transmission. However, to date there are no clinical trials with Reminyl in LBD to determine how well it actually works.

People with LBD are extremely sensitive to blocking the effects of the neurotransmitter dopamine. Antipsychotic medications, which block dopamine and are often given to combat the psychotic symptoms of LBD, may cause serious side effects, including severe rigidity and coma. Therefore, when psychosis is present it is essential to use the smallest possible dose of an antipsychotic medication. Because Seroquel (quetiapine) is about one hundred times less potent than the other antipsychotics, it is Dr. Shankle's treatment of choice when Exelon, Reminyl, and Aricept fail to control psychosis. If Seroquel does not control psychosis, then Geodon (ziprasidone) or low-dose Risperdal (risperidone) or low-dose Zyprexa (olanzapine) is the safest antipsychotic alternative for people with LBD.

Treating Movement Problems in LBD

Typically, physicians use dopamine-enhancing agents to treat movement problems in Parkinson's disease, such as muscle tremors and rigidity. Many physicians have found that increasing brain levels of dopamine to treat impaired movement in LBD works less well than in Parkinson's disease. The response to dopamine treatment is more variable in LBD than in Parkinson's disease, but when movement problems such as poor balance, falling, slowing down, and swallowing significantly impair function, then increasing dopamine is worth trying. Sometimes cholinesterase inhibitors themselves will cause movement problems as a side effect, in which case increasing brain dopamine can help.

There are several ways to increase brain dopamine. The most common way is to give Sinemet (carbidopa/levodopa), which increases the number of dopamine transmitter molecules in the brain. If this does not work, then movement can be improved by adding either Eldepryl (selegiline) or Comtan; both increase the amount of time the dopamine lasts before being degraded.

There are several potential side effects of these dopamine-increasing agents: abnormal movements become more likely after treatment for several years. The improved movement eventually wears off or may suddenly stop. Increasing dopamine levels can also cause or worsen psychosis.

Treating Mild Frontal-Temporal Lobe Dementia (FTLD)

At present, there is no known treatment that will delay the progression of FTLD. However, all causes of FTLD are believed to involve distortion of tau proteins, which form the neuron's skeleton or framework. It has therefore been proposed that agents that reduce this distortion will delay FTLD disease progression. One commonly prescribed medication that blocks excessive distortion of tau proteins is Depakote (valproic acid), an agent used in treating seizures and mood disorders. To date, there are no trials of Depakote in FTLD.

Recently, our research in applying the omentum to the brains of AD patients (see Chapter 9, page 207) resulted in a fortuitous finding that may lead to clues in treating FTLD. One patient's brain biopsy showed that he did not have AD but rather a type of FTLD called primary progressive aphasia. Within one month after surgery, this patient showed a marked improvement in ability to comprehend and respond to questions and complex tasks. His SPECT scan also started to show increases in brain activity that paralleled those seen in some of the AD patients who have undergone omental transposition surgery. While it is still too early to make any definite conclusions, this finding does open some interesting doors to research that could benefit people with FTLD.

Treating Symptoms in Mild FTLD

There are three classes of drugs to try with FTLD: antidepressants, cholinesterase inhibitors, and Namenda.

Antidepressants. The most effective treatments for the symptoms of FTLD have included agents that increase the neurotransmitters serotonin, dopamine, or norepinephrine. However, the response is often not dramatic. It may be that the reason these agents are helpful in FTLD is that they have primary effects on controlling mood-related behaviors such as aggression, agitation, and apathy. There are a number of different classes of these medications:

- Serotonin-enhancing medication, such as Prozac, Zoloft, Celexa, Lexapro, Luvox, and Paxil
- Norepinephrine-enhancing medications, such as Norpramin (desipramine)
- Dopamine-enhancing medications, such as Wellbutrin (bupropion)
- Dual or triaction medications, such as Effexor and Serzone

A trial of each of these agents is worthwhile in FTLD to see which type works best. High doses are often required. These medications are all considered to be different types of antidepressants and are discussed in the section on depressive pseudodementia.

Cholinesterase inhibitors. Trials of cholinesterase inhibitors in FTLD have been mostly unsuccessful, unless there is a mixed picture of FTLD with AD or VD.

Glutamate inhibitors (Namenda [Memantine]—an NMDA glutamate receptor blocker). Although Namenda has not been reported in treating FTLD, Dr. Shankle has treated a number of people with FTLD with Namenda and has obtained better results than he has seen with any other therapy. The real effect of Namenda ultimately depends on the balance between the excitation and inhibition in the frontal and temporal lobes. Namenda increases the overall excitation of the cortex, which can be quite helpful in people with rigidity, incoordination, difficulty performing complex tasks, speech, swallowing, and bladder control.

Treating Mild Head Trauma

As we discussed in Chapter 5, page 103, head injury is a significant risk factor for ADRD in the presence of the ApoE4 gene. One of the most important lessons we've learned through our brain imaging work is that brain injuries can be very significant, yet they are often overlooked. "Mild" brain injuries often have a greater effect than most people, including physicians, think that they do.

Traumatic brain injuries can cause physical difficulties such as severe headaches, dizziness, fatigue, and diminished motor skills. They also can create mental difficulties such as memory loss, difficulty with concentration, depression, hypersensitivity to noise, and photophobia (hypersensitivity to light). Often the most challenging problems for families to handle are the emotional and social difficulties that may arise after a traumatic brain injury, such as increased incidence of psychiatric problems, which is common even when the injury is relatively mild. A high percentage of those suffering even a mild concussion experience depression within the first two years following the injury. In addition, those with mild concussions experience an increased incidence of substance abuse, marital problems, and job-related problems, as well as incarceration and other legal problems.

It is interesting to note that many people forget that they have had significant brain injuries. Typically we ask patients five times during the course of their examinations whether or not they have had a significant brain injury. Many people say no, over and over again, and then "all of a sudden" remember a significant fall, car accident, or other significant trauma.

In treating mild head trauma we use antioxidants and ginkgo biloba to protect neurons from free radical damage and to increase blood flow to the brain. We also find it most effective to treat the brain systems involved in the injury. Of course, having a functional imaging study, such as a SPECT scan, helps to target treatment, because we can see which area or areas are affected. For prefrontal cortex problems—such as inattention, distractibility, disorganization, and low energy—we often use psychostimulants, such as Concerta or Adderall. When there are issues of decreased motivation, we use Provigil (modafanil) and Symmetrel (amantadine). For temporal lobe problems—such as mood instability, irritability, or aggression—we often use antiseizure medications, such as Neurontin, Depakote, or Lamictal. For deep limbic problems—such as depression, anxiety, or worrying—we often use antidepressants.

Treating Depressive Pseudodementia (DP)

As we have mentioned, depression can cause serious cognitive impairment and often masquerades as dementia. It is frequently overlooked and under-diagnosed. Depression is one of the most common illnesses in the United States and is estimated to affect 6 percent of the population at any point in time. Brain changes with depression affect areas involved with thinking and memory. Using preventive strategies for depression and treating it as early as possible is essential for helping to delay the cognitive problems associated with it.

Depression is clearly a biopsychosocial illness, which means it has genetic and biological causes, psychological causes (early childhood trauma and losses), and social causes (chronic stress from job, financial, or family problems). Depression needs to be treated in a biopsychosocial way.

Preventive Strategies for Depression

Know your risk. Depression runs in families. If you have the genetic vulnerability to depression, then prevention strategies are very important. Exercise and a proper diet are important prevention and early treatment strategies. In addition, work on your relationships. The better you get along with others, the better you will feel. One type of psychotherapy, called Interpersonal Psychotherapy (IPT), which teaches people how to get along better with others, was found to be an effective treatment for depression. Many community psychologists are trained in IPT.

Cognitive therapy, or therapy for your thoughts, has proven to be a very helpful tool in treating depression and anxiety disorders. What you allow to occupy your mind will sooner or later determine your feelings, your speech, and your actions. Every time you have a thought, your brain releases chemicals, myriad nerve transmissions go through your brain, and in a circular fashion you become aware of what you're thinking. Thoughts are real, and they have a real impact on how you feel and how you behave. Every time you have an angry, unkind, sad, or cranky thought, your brain releases negative chemicals that activate your deep limbic system and make your body feel bad. Think about how you felt the last time you were mad. When most people are angry their muscles become tense, their hearts beat faster, their hands start to sweat, and they may even begin to feel a little dizzy.

Every time you have a good thought, a happy thought, a hopeful thought, or a kind thought, your brain releases chemicals that calm your deep limbic system and help your body feel good. Think about how you felt the last time that you were happy. When most people are happy their muscles relax, their hearts beat slower, their hands become dry, and they breathe slower.

Mark George, M.D., demonstrated the brain's reaction to thought in an elegant study of brain function at the National Institutes of Mental Health. He studied the activity of the brain in 10 normal women under three different conditions. He studied these women when they were thinking neutral thoughts, happy thoughts, and sad thoughts. During the neutral thoughts, nothing changed in the brain. During happy thoughts, each woman demonstrated a cooling of her deep limbic system. During sad thoughts, each woman's deep limbic system became highly active.

Thoughts are powerful. They can make your mind and your body feel good, or they can make you feel bad. That is why emotional upset can manifest itself in physical symptoms, such as headaches or stomachaches. Your body is like an ecosystem. An ecosystem contains everything in the environment—the water, the land, the cars, the people, the animals, the vegetation, the houses, the landfills, and so on. A negative thought is like pollution to your system. Just as pollution in the Los Angeles Basin affects everyone who goes outdoors, so too do negative thoughts pollute your deep limbic system, your mind, and your body.

Thoughts are usually automatic, but they are not necessarily correct, nor do they always tell the truth. In fact, they often lie. Most of us believe our thoughts and do not know how to challenge them or direct them in a helpful way. The good news is that you can train your thoughts to be positive and hopeful or you can just allow them to be negative and upset you. Once you are aware of what you can do about your thoughts, you can choose to think good thoughts and feel good or you can choose to think bad thoughts and feel lousy. Through cognitive therapy, or thought therapy, you can learn how to change your thoughts and change the way you feel. One way to learn how to change your thoughts is to notice them when they are negative and talk back to them. If you think a negative thought without challenging it, your mind believes it and your body reacts to it. There are many wonderful cognitive therapists in the United States. See the website at www.amenclinic.com for a list of physicians and therapists in your area.

Early Interventions

The first treatment strategy for depression is to eliminate any of the obvious causes. Frequently medications, such as blood pressure or cancer medications, can cause depression. Notice the time frame of the onset of depression. If it is associated with any new medications, consult your physician for alternatives. Also make sure you get a good physical exam, and look for any medical problems that can cause depression, such as low thyroid function or pancreatic illness.

Proper diet and exercise are effective interventions. We have personally seen that the Zone Diet, recommended by Dr. Barry Sears, helps to enhance mood. In addition, one of the best natural treatments for depression is intense aerobic exercise, because it boosts blood flow to the brain, as well as energy levels.

When needed, medications or supplements are important treatments. It is important to point out that depression is not one disorder. As dementia has a variety of different causes and patterns, so does depression. In their recent book *Healing Anxiety and Depression*, Dr. Amen and the psychiatrist Lisa Routh explain that there are seven different types of depression and anxiety. They include anxiety because it occurs with depression nearly 70 percent of the time. Because each type has differing treatments, there is no one treatment that works effectively with all forms of depression. You may need to work with your doctor or health care professionals to find the right treatment and dosage for your particular situation.

Psychological interventions are a useful adjunct to effectively treat the entire spectrum of a depressive disorder. However, almost half a century of clinical medicine has shown that unless major depression is treated to correct the underlying biochemical deficiency in serotonin, norepinephrine, and possibly other neurotransmitters, psychological interventions on their own are ineffective.

Psychological interventions include psychotherapy, family therapy, and group therapy. Social therapies are also helpful, such as engaging in work or outside activities. Often loneliness seriously worsens depression or depressive tendencies, which is why many people appear more impaired when they go into long-term care facilities. Social interaction is essential, whether at church, the golf club, or family outings.

Prevention strategies and early intervention are important ways to keep dementia away for as long as possible, perhaps until we have even better prevention and treatment strategies.

chapter 9

Treatments for the Future

There is great hope for the future! Some very exciting treatments for Alzheimer's disease and related
disorders are in the pipeline. Until recently, preventing or curing ADRD
was considered a distant possibility. Our understanding of the underlying
biology of ADRD was simplistic and inadequate. Looking for a cure was
like navigating the ocean without even a sextant. Today, the picture is
bright. Through laboratory and population-based scientific studies supported by the National Institutes of Health and private foundations such
as the Alzheimer's Association, the Alzheimer's Research Foundation, the
Robert Wood Johnson Foundation, The John Douglas French Center, and
many others, physicians and scientists have discovered the genetic, behavioral, and environmental ADRD risk factors you have read about in this
book. Hope is created by action combined with a positive attitude that

supporting a search for the truth will lead to a better tomorrow. There is nothing haphazard about it.

The development and refinement of powerful imaging techniques, such as SPECT, PET, fMRI, and MRI, target anatomical and functional processes in the brain that are already giving us an improved ability to diagnose ADRD early. These techniques, along with better and more easily accessible annual screening methods (see Appendix A) can already help you and your doctor detect ADRD before symptoms develop or in their earliest and most treatable stage. This knowledge encourages prevention and treatment strategies long before ADRD impacts your life and the lives of those you care about most.

This chapter is organized according to how soon each approach is likely to be available—from very soon to later. The dates in parentheses give the year of expected availability.

Omental Transposition Surgery (OTS) (2004)

Over the last several years, we have been actively engaged in studying the effects of omental transposition surgery (OTS) in Alzheimer's disease. It is an exciting area of AD treatment research. The surgery involves implanting the omentum, a fatty tissue that covers the intestines in the abdomen with its blood vessels, up underneath the skin, and laying it directly

Figure 9.1. The Omentum in the Abdomen Lies Across the Intestines

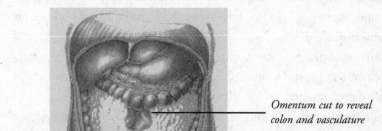

Omentum cut to reveal colon and vasculature

Omentum

onto the brain. The omentum is a very primitive tissue that is loaded with stem cells and growth factors. In observational studies, OTS has been helpful in a wide variety of neurological diseases, including Alzheimer's disease. However, until recently, it had never been rigorously scientifically evaluated.

The omental transposition surgery was pioneered by the surgeon Harry Goldsmith, who has been studying its use for over 30 years in patients with stroke, spinal cord resection, cerebral palsy, and Alzheimer's disease (79). During the 1960s, while working at Sloan Kettering Hospital in New York City, he discovered that the omentum helped speed wound healing in certain surgical patients. The idea came to him after he saw a woman who had a severely swollen arm after a mastectomy for breast cancer. In addition to removing the breast, mastectomies conducted years ago usually involved taking out the muscle on the chest wall (pectoralis muscle) and the lymphatic tissue in the armpit, which is essential for the arm's circulation. Arm swelling was a common side effect of extensive mastectomies. The woman's arm, Dr. Goldsmith described, was like dead weight for her, a large useless appendage hanging at her side. Eventually, her arm and shoulder were amputated. The thoughts of this woman's arm haunted him. As he thought about the fact that the surgery had damaged the lymphatics and blood supply in her armpit, he wondered what could be used to increase circulation and healing to the area. The thought came to him of draining the swelling using the omentum's extensive network of lymphatics and blood vessels.

Through animal laboratory research, Dr. Goldsmith found that he could dissect the omentum from the intestines, keep its blood supply attached, and implant it in other areas. Once laid onto these new areas, the omentum stimulated new blood vessels to grow, increased circulation, and released its transmitters, growth factors, and stem cells. A striking characteristic of omental tissue is that its arteries do not become hardened, even in people with hardened, atherosclerotic vessels.

In the late 1970s, Dr. Goldsmith implanted the omentum into stroke patients. According to Dr. Goldsmith, many improved, and more surgeries were done in the 1980s. He reported on a patient who had OTS 13 years after a stroke. The patient's neurological function improved, and it stayed improved. In 1984, Dr. Goldsmith reported that he had isolated an angiogenic (blood vessel–promoting) factor from the omentum. One injection causes new blood vessels to sprout. Dr. Goldsmith also found that the omentum increased choline acetyltransferase, the enzyme that catalyzes the reaction that creates acetylcholine in the brain, which is greatly reduced in AD and Lewy body disease. Over the past 30 years, a great deal of research has been done on the omentum to identify the stem cells, growth factors, and other chemicals it contains.

The omentum contains many nerves that control the gut. Those nerves, just like the ones in the brain, need nourishment and support. The omentum generates chemicals that nourish nerves and help them grow, and *it has been called a stem cell and growth factor factory.* The omentum also produces or enhances a wide range of neurotransmitters (such as acetylcholine, dopamine, norepinephrine, and serotonin). The omentum may

- Stimulate neurogenesis (make new neurons) (80)
- Stimulate synaptogenesis (make new connections) (81)
- Increase neurotransmitter activity (82)
- Enhance cell repair
- Reduce beta amyloid plaques (83)
- Block programmed cell death (84)

During OT surgery, the omentum is lifted off the intestines, while still remaining attached to its blood supply in the abdomen. It is then extended and tunneled underneath the skin of the chest and neck and placed directly onto the brain itself (Figure 9.2). The skull is then placed over the extended omentum, where it hopefully survives for two or more years to exert its effect. It is important to note that OTS is major surgery, opening up the abdomen to obtain the omentum and opening the skull to place the omentum over the brain and tunneling it under the skin of the chest and neck. There is potential for side effects, such as infection and pressure effects on the brain. The surgery should be done on people with ADRD who are otherwise healthy.

Figure 9.2. Omental Transposition Surgery

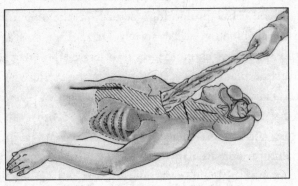

The omentum is carefully extended from the abdomen and placed onto the brain

Table 11.1 summarizes the clinical studies that have been done with OTS in a variety of neurological disorders. As you can see from the percentages of patients who have shown marked clinical improvement, OTS has a respectable track record in treating a number of diseases in which current treatments are either less effective or nonexistent. For example, over eight hundred patients with cerebral palsy, a disease with little to no treatment, have received OTS in China. Most of these patients have

Table 11.1. Neurological Disorders Treated with Omental Transposition			
Disorder	**Number of Patients**	**Percent Improved**	**Characterization of Improvement**
Cerebral palsy	800	80%	Walking, coordination, speech
Viral encephalitis	54	63%	Good improvement
Lack of oxygen at birth	125	94% 76% 68%	Functional skills Speech rate and clarity Muscle strength and tension
Stroke < 2 months before OTS	33	67%	Much improved speech and/or paralysis
Stroke > 2 months before OTS	22	50%	Much improved speech and/or paralysis
Alzheimer's disease (moderate to severe)	22	80%	Partial recovery that is clinically significant

markedly improved in their ability to function and greatly reduced the burden on their families. Fifty percent of persons with strokes that occurred more than two months before OTS showed clinical improvement. Percentages such as these are not to be scoffed at and deserve careful scientific research to understand what it is about the omentum that has such a powerful effect on brain diseases, regardless of whether their cause is lack of oxygen, blood flow, and perhaps even Alzheimer's disease.

One of the most intriguing findings about OTS in AD was reported by Dr. Normal Relkin, clinical director of New York Weill Cornell's Memory Disorders Program (83). In 1993, Dr. Goldsmith performed the first OTS in a man who had had Alzheimer's disease for about nine years at the time of surgery. At 10 months after surgery, his doctor reported his overall status was "remarkably improved," particularly in judgment, confusion, naming, and walking. A SPECT scan at that time showed brain activity increases of up to 100 percent in areas directly underneath the omentum, and smaller increases on the other side of the brain. Although the man died two and a half years later from unrelated causes, an autopsy showed that in the brain area directly in contact with the omentum, the number of beta amyloid laden plaques was greatly reduced. Elsewhere, the number of plaques was much higher. This plaque reduction resembles the effect of the so-called vaccines for AD, which in animal models of AD reverse the deficits seen in these animals. It is hoped that the rigorous scientific studies of OT surgery in AD patients currently underway will identify new treatments for AD that do not require surgery. Here are several examples of what has been seen in AD patients treated with OT surgery:

Stella ✢

Stella was a socially active individual until she developed AD about six years before she came to see Dr. Shankle. She had recently entered the moderate stage of AD and begun seeing her dead parents living in their house. Depression set in, her speech lessened, and she got angry at her husband, whom she no longer recognized and viewed as an intruder in their home. Medications partly helped control her depression, hallucinations, and agitation, but her behavior problems were so severe that she was unable to attend adult daycare, and her husband had to hire 24-hour home nursing. Aside from her behavioral and language problems, which are typical of moderate-stage AD, she was in good physical health. Her husband had heard about the omental transposition surgery, and after researching it, he decided that it was a better option than helplessly watching Stella deteriorate.

Stella's baseline SPECT study showed severe decreased activity in her temporal posterior parietal and frontal lobes, especially on the left side.

Stella's surgery lasted five hours, which is typical. Afterward, she stayed in the hospital for 10 days. Her husband was there with her, and he made sure she started eating and getting active as soon as it was practical, to avoid physical deterioration and to eliminate the intravenous lines and tube feedings that can cause infection after surgery.

Within several months, Stella no longer needed the antipsychotic medication she had required to control hallucinations. She also developed a brighter mood, and Dr. Shankle stopped her antidepressant medication. However, after several months, she became more irritable and depressed, which was reversed by restarting the antidepressant medication. Stella was also able to leave home and stay in adult daycare, which provided mental, physical, and social stimulation and gave her husband eight free hours a day. Her language and memory were still severely impaired, but she was able to socially communicate with others in a pleasant, friendly manner and could stay at home unattended for hours. Her husband felt he had gotten his wife back.

In the moderate and severe stages of AD, the mental abilities after OTS rarely show much improvement. Behavioral problems and functional abilities are more likely to improve. The omentum on Stella's brain was able to eliminate hallucinations and significantly improve social functioning in ways that medications had been unable to do.

The changes in brain activity over the 24 months after OT surgery were extraordinary. They clearly showed that the effect of the omentum was not simply to increase blood flow. Areas away from the omentum on both sides of the brain showed increases of 20 to 30 percent over the first year, beyond what had been accomplished in Stella by any of the treatments for Alzheimer's disease currently approved by the Food and Drug Administration.

Figures 9.3-4. Stella's Scans Before Treatment (Surface Views)

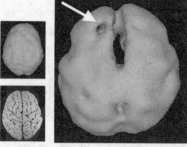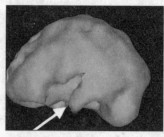

View from the top
Decreased frontal pole and
posterior parietal activity

Left side view
Decreased left frontal and
temporal lobe activity

Figures 9.5-6. Stella's Scans After OTS Treatment

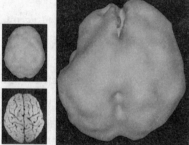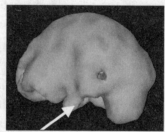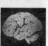

View from the top
Markedly increased
brain activity
(The dent on the left side is
the location of the omentum)

Left side view
Markedly increased brain activity
underneath omentum

It is important to note that Stella had a chronic, severe, degenerative illness, and according to her husband, she was rapidly deteriorating. The omental transposition surgery not only halted the progression of the illness for Stella but also gave her very significant improvements.

Jimmy ✣

Jimmy was a Shakespeare buff who developed Alzheimer's disease 10 years before coming to see Dr. Shankle. The most frustrating aspect of the disease for him was losing the ability to use language. He was more aware than many people with AD about the loss of his abilities, and he had started to decline sharply in the months prior to surgery. Jimmy and his wife heard about the omental transposition surgery on a CBS show that had interviewed Dr. Harry Goldsmith. Although Jimmy was moderately demented at the time of his surgery, he had relatively few behavioral problems, but he had severe language, memory, and visual problems. He was unable to comprehend simple sentences, and he used the same few words to respond to others. When shown a series of numbers, he had great difficulty recognizing them as numbers and tried to trace their shapes with his finger.

Jimmy's omentum was placed on the left side of his brain because the SPECT scan done at Dr. Amen's clinic showed a marked reduction in brain activity on the left side of the brain, particularly in areas affecting language. After surgery, Jimmy had a stormy course. He developed a series of infections from the intravenous and tube feeding lines, and he was hospitalized for almost a month. At one point, he was too weak to even get out of bed to go to the bathroom. Dr. Shankle started him on an intensive course of physical therapy to regain his strength, which helped and got him home. Over the next nine months, Jimmy's language began to improve. At one point, he came into Dr. Shankle's office and verbosely complained that he couldn't cite Shakespeare the way he used to!

Jimmy's scan provided an explanation for his improvement. His scan prior to surgery showed severe decreased activity of the left frontal and temporal lobes, which are the language areas of the brain. His subsequent scans have shown marked increased activity. At first the improvement was seen underneath the omentum, but later scans showed improvement in the brain at greater distances away from the omentum, even on the opposite side of the brain.

At Jimmy's last visit, he told Dr. Shankle that he was now taking a computer course that he was determined to succeed at. His motivation and judgment were improved, as was his outlook.

Figures 9.7-8. Jimmy's Scans Before OTS Treatment (Surface Views)

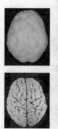
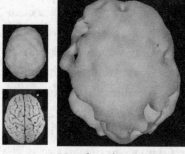
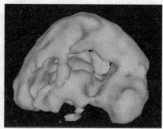
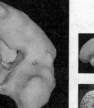
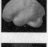
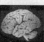

View from the top
Severe decreased left frontal
and occipital lobe activity

Left side view
Severe decreased left frontal
temporal, and occipital lobe
activity

Figures 9.9-10. Jimmy's Scans After OTS Treatment

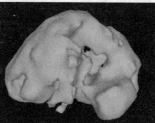
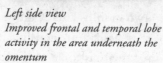

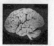

View from the top
Improved activity

Left side view
Improved frontal and temporal lobe
activity in the area underneath the
omentum

David ✣

David was a nuclear physicist who began to have trouble speaking at the age of 61. He was eventually diagnosed with Alzheimer's disease by a number of doctors. Six years into his illness, his daughter became very concerned because he had shown a noticeable decline within a few months and had hit one of the residents at his assisted living facility. Although he had become almost mute, he indicated to his daughter that if something couldn't be done, he wanted to die. When Dr. Shankle saw him, David was unable to understand how to perform any of the routine mental tests. His MRI and SPECT scans both showed greater damage in the left side of the brain, particularly the frontal and temporal lobes. While the diagnosis could have been a variant of Alzheimer's disease that affects language more than visual abilities, David could also have had primary progressive aphasia, a degenerative disease affecting the frontal and temporal lobes, particularly the left side. David's daughter decided that the omental surgery was her father's last hope.

David's surgery went remarkably well. His brain biopsy showed that he did not have AD but had findings consistent with frontal-temporal lobe dementia. He had some minor difficulties in the hospital but was discharged 12 days after surgery. David's daughter noted that within the first month, he became more alert and more spontaneous in his speech. Although his comprehension was still moderately to severely impaired, he understood more and more with the assistance of touch and visual cues, which had previously not helped.

Within two months after surgery, David was able to perform some of the mental tests he had previously failed to comprehend how to do. On several of the visual tasks, he obtained a perfect score. His daughter also noted that he started to use his address book for reminders and to look up names and other important information. He had forgotten how to use his address book almost a year prior to surgery. David also started walking to attend his favorite church daily. He had never walked to the church before.

The OTS stories offer much hope. At present, OTS for dementia is considered an experimental procedure. There is still much to learn, and the surgery may point the way to other exciting treatments.

Low-Pressure Shunts (2005)

These are devices that drain cerebrospinal fluid (CSF) from the brain to the abdominal cavity; CSF is a clear, salty fluid that completely surrounds the brain and spinal cord, both inside and out. It acts like a shock absorber for the brain and spinal cord; it bathes brain tissue in an ocean of fluid whose temperature and salt concentration stays constant, which makes it easier to control the brain's electrical activity, and it removes waste products from the brain, such as broken-down proteins, fats, and toxins.

Cerebrospinal fluid is produced from blood by specialized blood vessel structures, which act like a sieve to let the fluid in the blood through and keep out the red and white blood cells and large molecules. The resultant CSF, which looks like crystal-clear drinking water, contains the right balance of salts to allow nerve cells to efficiently generate electricity and do their job. The turnover of CSF declines with age. Hence it takes the brains of older persons longer to remove toxins. Since more free radicals also accumulate with age, because of lower cellular antioxidant levels, the slower CSF removal of free radicals makes damage to neurons even more likely.

A low-pressure shunt, marketed as COGNIShunt, is currently under investigation as a possible treatment for AD. The hypothesis is that beta amyloid, tau proteins, and other heavy molecular waste products ejected from brain cells and absorbed into the CSF are more likely to drop out of a slowly moving, low-pressure stream of ventricular fluid, and be captured by the shunt tube, which deposits them into the abdominal cavity. Preliminary studies show that it is more effective in clearing tau proteins than beta amyloid from AD brains. Because tau protein abnormalities also occur in frontal temporal lobe dementia and are thought to be harmful, it may be a useful treatment for this group of diseases. However, the manufacturers are currently testing it for AD only. The risk of infection is similar to that of other types of shunts: about 10 percent.

In October 2002 the journal *Neurology* reported the results of the early studies on COGNIShunt. In the study, 15 participants were selected to receive the shunt, and 14 people received no investigational treatment. All participants had been diagnosed with mild to moderate Alzheimer's disease. Subjects were followed for one year. The primary objective of the pilot study was to assess the safety of the shunt procedure. Side effects among the 15 people receiving the surgical treatment included seizures (two participants), shunt infection (one), small injury in the abdomen during surgery (one), severe postoperative headache (one), postoperative pain (eight), nausea (seven), headache (five), abdominal pain (five), and blockage in a shunt (three).

Neuropsychological testing was done every three months. The researchers noted a trend that symptoms were stabilized in people who received the treatment and that there was a decline in people who did not receive treatment. Although the sample is too small to draw conclusive conclusions, it does offer hope, and points to the need for further research. In a real sense, if low-pressure shunts are helpful, they could offer hope to treat a variety of neurologic diseases in which heavy molecules cause brain damage. Such conditions include frontal-temporal lobe dementia, Lewy body disease, Parkinson's disease, and others. For information about the ongoing studies being performed by the manufacturer, Eunoe, e-mail info@eunoe-inc.com or phone (888) 4MY-MIND or (888) 469-6463.

Genetic Hope for the Future (2005)

The Human Genome Project has already identified dozens of genes that can affect your risk for developing dementia or can determine how you will respond to certain medications. Someday you will be able to identify your genetic risks *and modify them if you choose* before the disease is clinically apparent. The simplest example of this is that your cholesterol level is 90 percent controlled by your genes, but you can lower your cholesterol through diet, exercise, and the proper medication. The situation with ADRD is no different (in fact, high cholesterol is one of the risk factors for ADRD).

Genetic Testing

As we mentioned earlier, we believe people should be allowed to make a thoughtful decision about apoliproteinE genotype testing. There are legitimate reasons for wanting to know if you or other family members are at risk. If they have the ApoE4gene, then they should avoid activities that put them at risk for a brain injury and take advantage of prevention and early screening measures.

Vaccines (2008)

A recent development in the treatment of AD is vaccination. Throughout history, vaccines have been employed to treat infectious diseases such as smallpox. Vaccines work because the body's immune system responds against foreign substances it has encountered before. Essentially, a vaccine is a part of a bacterium, virus, or other organism that is foreign to your body. The first time your immune cells encounter one of these "foreigners," they make antibodies—proteins that attack and kill the invading organism to keep you from dying. Your immune cells are like elephants—they never forget. If the same foreign organism invades your body sometime in the future, the immune cells floating around in your bloodstream (the white blood cells) will "recognize" the invader and produce the right antibodies to kill it.

In theory, vaccination could halt or slow progression of AD by enabling the body to recognize beta amyloid plaques as "brain invaders." By giving small amounts of a beta amyloid vaccine, a person's immune system could be activated to produce antibodies to attack and remove the beta amyloid from the brain. This has been accomplished in mouse models, genetically engineered to overproduce beta amyloid. By the time these mice reach adulthood, they are "demented." For example, they get lost and can't find their way to recently learned favorite food locations. The first vaccine for human AD, named AN-1792, was developed by neurobiologists at a small biotech company called Elan Pharmaceuticals. It was made from the beta amyloid protein. Animal studies performed in 1999 and published in the journal *Nature* confirmed that injections of AN-1792 blocked accumulation of beta amyloid plaques in one of the mouse models of AD. If these mice were injected with AN-1792, they wouldn't get lost, indicating better spatial short-term memory.

These promising results prompted the Food and Drug Administration to approve Phase I clinical trials to assess the safety and tolerability of the vaccine in humans. Elan and Wyeth-Ayerst Laboratories conducted the first Phase I study involving one hundred subjects with mild to moderate AD. The results were very promising. The vaccine did not cause significant adverse side effects in any of the subjects, and many displayed a positive immune response, causing antibody levels to rise.

Given the success of Phase I, Elan and Wyeth-Ayerst Laboratories moved into the second phase of clinical trials and in 2001 enrolled 375 subjects with mild to moderate AD. Among those subjects, three hundred were assigned to AN-1792 treatment and the rest received a placebo. In January 2002, however, Elan suspended the study when four of the subjects receiving AN-1792 exhibited inflammation of the brain and spinal cord and died. After 11 more subjects showed similar inflammation, the study was halted altogether.

Presumably, the AN-1792 vaccine stimulated antibodies that not only attacked beta amyloid but also attacked normal brain tissue to produce inflammation and sometimes death. Further clarification of what happened was given by Christoph Hock, M.D., in the October 2002 issue of *Nature Medicine,* which examined 30 of the subjects from the Phase IIA clinical trials. He and his colleagues determined that vaccinated subjects did make antibodies to beta amyloid after receiving several doses of AN-1792. Although quantities of antibodies differed among subjects, the level of antibody did not dictate whether or not a person acquired brain inflammation.

Since the AN-1792 failure, many companies around the globe have been working to develop a beta amyloid vaccine that will not attack normal brain tissue. New strategies include altering the size of the beta amyloid fragments in the vaccine so that a less vigorous immune response occurs or administering antibodies that have been genetically altered. One of these companies will certainly succeed in producing a safe vaccine for humans. Once beta amyloid is successfully cleared from the brains of persons with Alzheimer's disease, we will better understand how much beta amyloid causes the dysfunction of AD.

The development of a vaccine should not lead you to think that you can detect AD at any stage in the disease and simply reverse it with a vaccine. There is much brain damage associated with the accumulation of beta amyloid that will not be reversed. Therefore, just like high blood pressure and diabetes, it still makes the most sense to detect AD and related disorders as early as possible to minimize the damage.

Growth Factors (2008)

Over the next decade, growth factors will become standard therapy in treating brain diseases. Growth factors are what help the brain develop, mature, and repair itself when damaged. By selectively manipulating one or more of the growth factors in persons with various brain diseases, it will be possible to obtain functional recovery never dreamed possible.

A major issue with all growth factors is getting them into the brain. If swallowed, growth factors are digested before they get into the bloodstream. If injected directly into the blood, very little of the growth factors can get into the brain, because they are too large to cross the blood-brain barrier. The same problem occurs if they are inhaled through the lungs.

However, Dr. William H. Frey II, director of one of the oldest Alzheimer's centers in the United States, has discovered an intranasal method of bypassing the blood-brain barrier to effectively deliver growth factors and other Alzheimer's therapeutic agents to the brain. Dr. Frey began his research back in the 1970s. To date, he and other researchers have demonstrated effective delivery of a large variety of molecules through the nose, including estrogen, insulin-like growth factor 1, fibroblastic growth factors, vasoactive intestinal peptide (VIP), insulin, and the hormone that controls cortisol (CRH) (85). Intranasal delivery of FGF-2 or of EGF has even demonstrated new neuron formation in the adult mouse brain (86).

Nerve growth factor. In the 1980s, researchers learned that administering a protein molecule called nerve growth factor (NGF) to older rats that exhibited memory impairment during a maze trial improved their ability to negotiate the maze. Nerve growth factor promotes regeneration of damaged nerve cells that contain the neurotransmitter acetylcholine and promotes growth of the axons and dendrites of these cholinergic neurons to reconnect to other nerve cells. Because cholinergic neurons are heavily damaged by AD, the discovery that NGF improves the memory of older rats inspired neuroscientists to investigate its therapeutic potential.

Nerve growth factor gene therapy was developed to reduce disease progression by delivering growth factors to regions of the brain where cholinergic neurons and their connections (synapses) are dying. This therapy has been shown to reduce and prevent the death of additional cholinergic neurons. Furthermore, NGF gene therapy has been safely delivered to primates.

Cerebrolysin is an example of an NGF drug that is showing promise in improving mental function, in studies outside of the United States. The results of a recent clinical study of Cerebrolysin were recently reported in the journal *Clinical Drug Investigation*. Cerebrolysin is manufactured by Ebewe Pharmaceuticals of Austria and is currently approved for marketing in 28 countries but not yet in the United States. Dr. Xiao Shifu of the Shanghai Mental Health Center in China and his colleagues in the Cerebrolysin Study Group compared the effects of Cerebrolysin with those of a placebo in 157 patients with mild to moderate Alzheimer's disease. The drug was given intravenously five days a week for four weeks. The findings showed that Cerebrolysin improved measures of mental function and possibly functional activities more than placebo. Side effects reported by patients receiving Cerebrolysin were temporary and mild, and ranged from a feeling of heat to agitation to hypersensitivity reactions. Clinical research on the drug will continue with the aim of obtaining marketing approval in the United States and other countries.

Other growth factors that may be used for AD therapy include insulin-like growth factor 1 and epidermal growth factor—which generate new neurons in the adult mammalian brain—plus brain-derived neurotrophic factor (BDNF) and neurotrophin-3, which promote neuronal cell survival. By promoting new neuron formation and combating neuronal cell death and shrinkage, future treatment with growth factors should provide major improvements in the treatment of AD and other brain disorders.

Generating New Neurons (2009)

Stem cells and TGF alpha. Brain stem cell therapy encourages very versatile cells to develop into neurons to replace damaged or diseased cells. Considered one of the most promising frontiers of science, stem cell research could lead to life-saving therapies for AD, Parkinson's disease, diabetes, heart disease, stroke, and spinal cord injuries. Stem cell research is in its infancy and is still considered very controversial because one source of stem cells comes from early-stage human embryos. Some antiabortion groups call stem cell research morally unacceptable because the embryonic stem cells come from embryos that have been aborted. However, we now know that stem cells can be made in a variety of ways that do not require human embryos. Scientists working in the last few years with private funding, primarily from the company Geron, isolated stem cells from aborted fetuses and unused embryos from infertility treatments. They successfully multiplied them in laboratories, creating a supply for research purposes. The National Institutes of Health, the most significant funder of U.S. medical research, says these lab-grown stem cells do not constitute embryos. Therefore, this federal agency can legally fund experiments using the cells.

Stem cells are the basic or primordial cells from which all of a human's tissues and organs develop. By themselves, the cells can't grow into a human being. But if scientists can learn how the cells switch on to form different organs and tissues, they might be able to grow heart cells to rebuild disease-ravaged hearts, insulin-producing cells for diabetics, or brain cells for victims of neurologic and psychiatric diseases.

Human embryonic stem cells emerge five to seven days into an embryo's development, when the embryo is a hollow sphere of as few as eight cells. The sphere consists of an outer layer of cells, which goes on to form the placenta, and an inner cluster of cells, known as the inner cell mass, which goes on to form all of the tissues of the body. At this stage, the embryo is known as a blastocyst. Embryonic stem cells arise from the inner cell mass. They have the potential to differentiate, or specialize, into each of the body's two hundred tissue types, such as heart cells, bone cells, cartilage cells, liver cells, and even brain cells.

By exposing stem cells to certain growth factors, scientists have succeeded in prompting the cells to differentiate in the laboratory into specific types of cells. However, researchers have much to learn about how to grow and maintain such differentiated cells at a stage in their development that would make them useful for treating diseases.

Although the prospect of using stem cells to treat disease shows great potential, there are major problems regarding its practical use. Not only is the tissue severely limited in supply, it is also quite vulnerable and easily contaminated. The body's immune system may reject introduced stem cells because they are foreign substances. Genetically engineered stem cells have higher rates of DNA mutation and can transform into cancer cells. Surgical procedures to introduce stem cells may be difficult to perform. How to target stem cells to replace just the ones that died and not other types of cells could be very tricky and difficult.

Yet progress is being made. In an article by Bruce Goldman in *Signal* magazine, Martin McGlynn, the president and CEO of StemCells, Inc., says: "We've identified the central-nervous-system stem cell, purified it, expanded it, transplanted it, and shown that it engrafts, migrates, and differentiates into all three major brain-cell types." So far, there's been no spontaneous tumor formation yet in over one thousand mice tested, McGlynn says.

Another promising area of progress comes from our colleague, the neuroanatomist Dr. James Fallon, at the University of California, Irvine. He and his colleagues identified the amino acid compound called transforming growth factor alpha, or TGF-alpha. This growth factor plays an important role in embryonic development and may be the first growth factor that affects an embryo; TGF-alpha is produced in endothelial cells, which are found in the linings of organs and tissues such as the intestines and blood vessels, and encourages stem cell proliferation. "It's kind of a handy, all-use growth factor," says Dr. Fallon. Levels of TGF-alpha increase in the area of the brain responsible for Parkinson's patients as the disease worsens. This suggests that TGF-alpha may be involved in tissue repair or cell replacement.

The presence of TGF-alpha in the brain may explain why careful studies of the numbers of neurons in the brains of severely demented AD patients have only found four brain areas that actually have a reduced number of neurons; TGF-alpha may be stimulating new neuron formation to replace dying neurons in most brain areas. However, the areas hit hardest by AD (the hippocampus and entorhinal cortex), simply cannot replace all the neurons that have died and consequently show reduced neuron number.

Several companies have unsuccessfully tried other stem cells or growth factors in clinical trials. Dr. Fallon says TGF-alpha is different. He commented, "Other growth factors don't work nearly as well as TGF-alpha does. You may get a couple of cells here or there with these, but it's transitory, very light. What you see when you inject TGF-alpha into the damaged brain is nothing like what anybody else has ever reported. We were seeing *millions* of cells." So TGF-alpha seems to have great potential.

As you can see, the coming years offer many exciting new developments in the field of Alzheimer's disease, dementia, and aging. These new therapies will have potentially greatest value to those who detect problems early so that complex disease-related changes are halted or minimized before they produce irreversible brain damage.

chapter 10

For Caregivers and Their Families: Resources

❧ Dementia is a family problem. It affects the person and her spouse, children, grandchildren, neighbors, and friends. The stress among family members is often staggering. Caregivers often die before their affected loved one because they ignore their own health needs and are under severe, chronic stress.

Put On Your Own Oxygen Mask First

One of the major worries of family members is their own risk for dementia. Since many of the risk factors for ADRD have strong genetic underpinnings, family members are usually at increased risk. When you add chronic stress to genetic risk, and then neglect your own health needs, the risk for problems can dramatically increase. Taking care of oneself is critical to being able to help the affected family member. Self-care is akin to what flight attendants say to us on airplanes before takeoff: "If the cabin pressure drops and oxygen masks come down, put your mask on first, before you put the masks on for others." You have to take care of yourself if you are to be at your best to care for others.

Assess your own risk, and take prevention steps as early as possible. Fifteen percent or more of caregiver spouses also have dementia that goes undetected and untreated because they neglect their own healthcare needs. It is extremely difficult to effectively care for someone else when you are also experiencing a dementing illness. It is hard to remember to give medication on time, properly feed your loved one, oversee proper hygiene needs, control your own temper when irritated (which can happen frequently), and give enough positive stimulation. Make sure you have your own medical appointments, eat and exercise properly, take the supplements and medications you need, and have a confidant to bounce off frustrations and ideas. DO NOT FEEL GUILTY FOR TAKING CARE OF YOURSELF! It is essential if you are going to be effective in caring for your loved one.

Sam and Patty

When they came to the Amen Clinic, Sam and Patty were 74 and 71. Patty was a diabetic who had had a stroke the previous year and was having problems with recovery. She also complained of memory problems, which were obvious to her family members. Sam, her husband of 48 years, was Patty's caregiver. He took care of her meals, diabetes, medications, doctor appointments, and physical therapy rehab sessions. Sam was having trouble managing all the details. In addition, he had problems with his temper and was frequently frustrated with Patty. They came to the clinic primarily for Patty's problems. Sam was evaluated only at his daughter's insistence after she saw how rough Sam could be with her mom.

To everyone's surprise, Sam's brain appeared to be much more impaired than Patty's. Her brain showed the obvious stroke in the back of her right brain, but otherwise there was good activity. Sam's brain showed a patchy pattern of severely decreased activity over many brain areas. Sam had played football in school and had drunk heavily until he was in his forties. Both were demented—Patty with vascular dementia and Sam with what appeared to be a dementia due to a combination of football-related repeated brain injuries and prior alcohol abuse. We optimized Patty's vascular dementia treatment by tightly controlling her diabetes, starting Reminyl, alpha lipoic acid, and vitamins C and E and continuing her baby aspirin. We treated Sam's traumatic-alcoholic dementia by starting alpha lipoic acid, vitamin C and E, and Namenda (memantine). Within several months they both improved.

Because of limited funds, caregivers often spend their resources on the "obviously" affected person and scrimp on themselves. As you can see from the story of Patty and Sam, this is a bad idea. You need to be healthy to care for those you love, and neglecting yourself is a poor model for your family to see. With limited resources, balance your needs with needs of the person under your care.

Caregivers spend an average of 12 hours per day, or 84 hours a week, taking care of their loved one! No wonder psychiatric symptoms of depression and anxiety are so common. Who wouldn't be stressed out working two full-time jobs and not getting paid? Dr. Shankle's online depression screen (see Appendix A) has been used to check for depression in family caregivers and has found that 80 percent of them fit the diagnosis of major depression. The traditional psychological explanation for depression is experiencing loss. Caregivers experience many, many losses, such as the loss of a job from having to care for the person at home, loss of emotional support from their loved one, financial losses, and loss of independence. Caregivers often complain of losing the personality of their loved one. "He is not the same person" is a common statement. Anxiety is also a very common caregiver problem. Anxiety comes from chronic worry about the affected person, worry about one's own risk, and the chronic stress of having to supervise another person.

Regardless of the cause of depression or anxiety, treating these conditions greatly improves the health of caregivers and of those they care for. Chronic feelings of sadness, trouble sleeping, panic attacks, change in appetite, weight gain or loss, or just not being able to "shake the blues" are all symptoms that should be evaluated and treated. Make sure to get evaluated, see your doctor, and/or see a counselor. Counseling and medication can be of great benefit during this difficult time.

Caregivers who are raising children and caring for their demented par-

Figures 10.1-2. Patty's Scans–Stroke Right Side

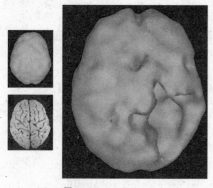
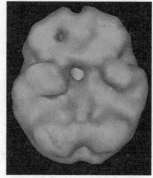
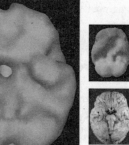

Top view
Decreased right hemisphere

Underside view
Decreased left temporal lobe
activity

Figures 10.3-4. Sam's Scan–Overall Decreased Activity

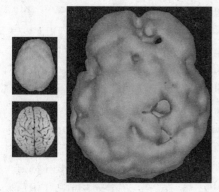
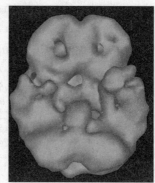
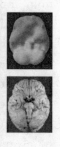
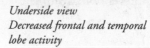

Top view
Overall decreased activity

Underside view
Decreased frontal and temporal
lobe activity

ents while trying to build their careers belong to the "sandwich generation." These responsible, caring people suffer extraordinary feelings of guilt, depression, anxiety, resentment, and anger over being squeezed from all sides. They neglect their own needs, their marriages are severely strained, sometimes leading to divorce, and friendships are left behind. Sandwich generation caregivers may also experience midlife crisis as they face the reality of their own eventual death through loss of family and close friends. A midlife crisis raises many questions, such as: "Is this how I want to live the rest of my life?" If you are unhappy with life and your parent needs constant attention, it can set up an emotional conflict that negatively affects the whole family.

Caring for People with Dementia

Learn as much about dementia as possible. Robert Pasnau, M.D., past president of the American Psychiatric Association, said that coping requires three things: information, self-esteem, and a sense of control. Obtaining accurate information is the critical first step in coping with dementia. The more accurate information you have, the more likely you are to get the best help. The national Alzheimer's Association's website is an invaluable resource (www.alz.org). Dr. Shankle's website (www.PreventAD.org) contains practical knowledge about each of the causes of dementia so that caregivers will better understand what they are dealing with.

Obtaining support for yourself, your family, and the affected person is critical. Many caregivers feel isolated and alone. A sense of relief can come from knowing other people who have similar problems or deal with similar situations. In addition, interacting with other families affected by dementia can give you more ideas on coping strategies for specific situations. There are many ways to get emotional support for Alzheimer's disease and related dementias. Alzheimer's Association is a great resource. In addition, they have local chapters where you can attend meetings, get information, and learn the latest information.

Caregivers need care too. Here is a list of resources to help you learn more about prevention, treatment, and caring for those affected by ADRD.

Organizations

Several organizations offer helpful information about Alzheimer's disease and related disorders (ADRD). To learn more about support groups, services, research, and additional publications, you may wish to contact the following:

Alzheimer's Association
225 North Michigan Avenue, fl. 17
Chicago, IL 60611-1676

1-800-272-3900
web address: www.alz.org

This nonprofit association supports families and caregivers of patients with ADRD. Almost 300 chapters nationwide provide referrals to local resources and services and sponsor support groups and educational programs. Online and print versions of publications are also available at the website.

Alzheimer's Disease Education and Referral (ADEAR) Center
P.O. Box 8250
Silver Spring, MD 20907-8250
1-800-438-4380
301-587-4352 (fax)
web address: www.alzheimers.org

This service of the National Institute on Aging is funded by the federal government. It offers information and publications on diagnosis, treatment, patient care, caregiver needs, long-term care, education and training, and research related to AD. Staff members answer telephone and written requests and make referrals to local and national resources. Publications and videos can be ordered through the ADEAR Center or via the website.

Children of Aging Parents
1609 Woodbourne Road, Suite 302A
Levittown, PA 19057-1511
1-800-227-7294
web address: www.caps4caregivers.org

This nonprofit group provides information and materials for adult children caring for their older parents. Caregivers of people with Alzheimer's disease also may find this information helpful.

Eldercare Locator
1-800-677-1116
web address: www.eldercare.gov

The Eldercare Locator is a nationwide directory assistance service helping older people and their caregivers locate local support and resources for older Americans. It is funded by the Administration on Aging (AoA), which also provides a caregiver resource called *Because We Care—A Guide for People Who Care*. The AoA Alzheimer's Resource Room contains information for families, caregivers, and professionals about AD, caregiving, working with and providing services to people with AD, and where you can turn for support and assistance.

Family Caregiver Alliance (FCA)
690 Market Street, Suite 600
San Francisco, CA 94104
415-434-3388
web address: www.caregiver.org

Family Caregiver Alliance is a community-based nonprofit organization offering support services for those caring for adults with AD, stroke, traumatic brain injuries, and other cognitive disorders. Programs and services include an information clearinghouse for the FCA's publications.

The National Institute on Aging (NIA) Information Center
P.O. Box 8057
Gaithersburg, Maryland 20898-8057
1-800-222-2225
301-589-3014 (fax)
web address: www.nia.nih.gov

The NIA offers a variety of types of information about health and aging, including the Age Page series and the NIA Exercise Kit, which contains an 80-page exercise guide and 48-minute closed-captioned video. Caregivers can find many Age Pages on the website.

The Simon Foundation for Continence
Box 815
Wilmette, IL 60091
1-800-237-4666
web address: www.simonfoundation.org

This foundation helps individuals with incontinence, their families, and the health professionals who provide their care. The foundation provides books, pamphlets, tapes, self-help groups, and other resources.

Well Spouse Foundation
63 W. Main Street, Suite H
Freehold, NJ 07728
1-800-838-0879
web address: www.wellspouse.org

Well Spouse is a nonprofit membership organization that gives support to wives, husbands, and partners of the chronically ill and/or disabled. It publishes the bimonthly newsletter *Mainstay.*

Alzheimer's Prevention Foundation International
2420 N. Pantano Road
Tucson, AZ 85715
520-749-8374
www.AlzheimersPrevention.org

Conducts research and provides educational programs.

Further Reading

The 36-Hour Day: A Family Guide to Caring for Persons with Alzheimer Disease, Related Dementing Illnesses, and Memory Loss in Later Life, by Nancy L. Mace and Peter V. Rabins. Warner Books, 2001.

Change Your Brain, Change Your Life, by Daniel G. Amen. Three Rivers Press, 2000.

Elder Rage, or Take My Father . . . Please!: How to Survive Caring for Aging Parents, by Jacqueline Marcell. Impressive Press, 2001.

Mayo Clinic on Alzheimer's Disease, Ronald C. Petersen M.D., editor. Kensington, 2002.

The Memory Bible: An Innovative Strategy for Keeping Your Brain Young, by Gary Small. Hyperion, 2002.

Saving Your Brain: The Revolutionary Plan to Boost Brain Power, Improve

Memory, and Protect Yourself Against Aging and Alzheimer's, by Jeff Victoroff. Doubleday, 2002.

The Omega Diet; The Lifesaving Nutritional Program Based on the Diet of the Island of Crete, by Artemis P. Simopoulos, M.D., and Jo Robinson. Perennial, 1999.

The Zone and *The Omega Rx Zone,* by Barry Sears. Regan Books, 2003.

PreventAD.com

Dr. Shankle and his wife, Junko, a dedicated Alzheimer's researcher, have personally funded and devoted seven unpaid years of their lives to build an effective solution to Alzheimer's Disease and Related Disorders (ADRD). They and their team of computer and medical scientists, healthcare and business professionals, plus ADRD patients and their loved ones, have built tools to help prevent or delay ADRD by an average of six to seven years, which reduces its total cost by $100,000 to $300,000. These tools have already helped thousands of families and individuals affected by ADRD, and are available to the public on the worldwide web at www.PreventAD.org. A more comprehensive version for healthcare professionals is available at www.mccare.com.

These tools—the Mental Skills Test, the Memory Screen, the Depression Screen, and the Health Monitoring System—grew out of research initially supported by grants from the Alzheimer's Association, and provide cutting-edge ADRD knowledge for public and professionals. They are confidential, fully automated and interactive, accurate yet brief, and generate immediate results with detailed reports for both patient/family and physician.

The Mental Skills Test (MST) directly tests an individual's mental abilities—memory, mental speed, attention, judgment, and language—in about 10 minutes, and is 97 percent accurate in detecting the earliest stages of ADRD, which can be as early as eight years before ADRD is typically diagnosed. There is online training that takes a few minutes to learn how to give the MST, and it is equally accurate when given by a medical office worker compared with a professional neuropsychologist. When used by families to test their loved ones, it is useful to confirm the test by having it repeated at their doctor's office.

The Memory Screen (MS) asks a series of questions about an individual's memory, reasoning, and other mental abilities, and uses advanced computer science methods—similar to those used by NASA scientists to explore the universe—to recognize patterns of answers that detect the earliest stages of ADRD with 94 percent accuracy. The highest accuracy is obtained when someone who knows an individual well takes the MS for them. However, persons who are good self judges can take the MS for themselves. The MS combined with the MST can distinguish impairments that are likely to get worse from those that are not. The MS is also helpful when you are concerned about someone who is unwilling to be evaluated for a memory problem or for ADRD.

The Depression Screen (DS) asks a series of questions to help determine whether someone has major depression as defined by the American Psychiatric Association. The DS also evaluates the effectiveness of antidepressants being taken, and when appropriate, provides recommendations to adjust ineffective antidepressant therapy. When the MST indicates that depression could cause the observed findings, the DS can evaluate that possibility. The DS can also be taken for an individual by someone who knows him or her well.

The Health Monitoring System (HMS) is an interactive tool that allows families or individuals to track over forty of the most common problems associated with ADRD and other brain disorders. It also allows them to include any other medical problems that exist. The HMS can be extraordinarily helpful to a physician—whose time is limited—to allow him to get a complete picture of the situation, so it can be better managed.

As a purchaser of this book, you are entitled to one free Memory Screen at www.PreventAD.com. When you visit this website, you will see a section reviewing the contents of this book. Within that section, you will find a green icon for a free Memory Screen. Clicking the icon will guide you through a registration process and you will be prompted to enter the following registration code: PAD-1-FMS. This free offer is available for a limited time.

How to Find the Help
You Need

When is it time to see a professional about memory problems? We recommend that people seek professional help for themselves or a family member when problems start. The earlier you get help, the more likely preventive interventions are to work. If you are experiencing persistent memory issues, or others notice your memory problems, then it's time to get help. If your problems are interfering with your ability to function, at home or at work, it is urgent that you get help. Pride can get in the way of seeking a proper diagnosis. People want to be strong and rely on themselves, and no one wants to believe there is a problem. We are constantly reminded of the strength it takes to make the decision to get help. And getting help should be looked at as a way to get your brain operating at its full capacity.

What do I do when a loved one is in denial about needing help? Unfortunately, many people who have early signs of dementia do not see the problems. People do not want to be seen as stupid or defective and do not seek help until they (or their loved ones) can no longer avoid the problems. Men are especially affected by denial. Many men, when faced with obvious problems in their jobs or families, refuse to see the problems. Their lack of awareness and strong tendency toward denial prevent them from seeking help until more damage than necessary has been done.

Dr. Amen dealt with this very serious issue in his family. One of his close relatives, William, 68, who had a history of alcoholism, brain injury, and diabetes, started to show signs of trouble. He forgot appointments, stumbled over finding words, and started to get lost and confused when driving. He became angry and frustrated when someone pointed out the problems. He made many excuses for the problems, including having low blood sugar or not getting enough sleep. Dr. Amen was called by the family to intervene. He sat down with William, gave a clear description of the problems, and encouraged William to get a SPECT scan. The scan showed serious evidence of problems, especially in the temporal lobes, parietal lobes, and prefrontal cortex. Seeing evidence of the problem, William agreed to get help, which included Aricept, Wellbutrin, a stimulating antidepressant, ginkgo biloba, vitamins E and C, and baby aspirin. Within a month he was much improved.

Here are several suggestions to help people who are unaware or unwilling to get the help they need.

1. *Try the straightforward approach* first (but with a new brain twist). Clearly tell the person what concerns you. Tell the person that the problems may be due to underlying brain patterns that can be tuned up. Tell the person that help may be available—help not to cure a defect but rather help to optimize how the brain functions. Tell the person you know he or she is trying to do his or her best, but the problems may be getting in the way of success. Emphasize improved access to the brain, not defect.
2. *Give information.* Books, videos, and articles on the subjects you are concerned about can be of tremendous help. Many people come to see

us because they read a book, saw a video, or read an article. Good information can be very persuasive, especially if it is presented in a positive, life-enhancing way.

3. When a person remains resistant to help, even after you have been straightforward and given good information—*plant seeds.* Plant ideas about getting help and then water them regularly. Drop an idea, article, or other information about the topic from time to time. If you talk too much about getting help, people become resentful and will refuse to get help just to spite you.

4. *Protect your relationship with the person.* People are more receptive to people they trust than to people who nag and belittle them. Work on gaining the person's trust over the long run. It will make the person more receptive to your suggestions. Do not make getting help the only thing you talk about. Make sure you are interested in the person's whole life, not just his or her potential medical appointments.

5. *Give new hope.* Many people with these problems have tried to get help and it did not work or it even made them worse. Educate the person on new brain technology that helps professionals be more focused and more effective in treatment efforts.

How do I find a competent professional who uses this new brain science thinking? We get many calls, faxes, and e-mails a week from people all over the world looking for competent professionals in their area who think along the lines of the principles outlined in this book. Because this approach is on the edge of what is new in brain science, other professionals may be hard to find. However, finding the right professional for evaluation and treatment is critical to the healing process. The right professional can have a very positive impact on your life; the wrong professional can make things worse. There are a number of steps to take in finding the best person to assist you.

1. *Get the best person you can find.* Saving money up front may cost you in the long run. The right help is not only cost-effective but saves unnecessary pain and suffering. Don't only rely on a person who is on your managed care plan. That person may or may not be a good fit for

you. Search for the best. If he or she is on your insurance plan—great. But don't let that be the primary criterion.

2. *Use a specialist.* Diagnosis and treatment for memory problems are expanding at a rapid pace. Specialists keep up with the details in their fields, while generalists (family physicians) have to try to keep up with everything. If we had a heart arrhythmia, we would see a cardiologist rather than a general internist. We want someone to treat us who has seen hundreds or even thousands of cases like ours.

3. Once you get the names of competent professionals, *check their credentials.* Very few patients ever check a professional's background. Board certification is a positive credential. To become board-certified, physicians have had to pass additional written and verbal tests. They have had to discipline themselves to gain the skill and knowledge that are acceptable to their colleagues.

4. *Set up an interview* with the professional to see whether or not you want to work with him or her. Generally you have to pay for their time, but it is worth spending time getting to know the people you will rely on for help.

5. *Read the work of or hear the professional speak,* if possible. Many professionals write articles or books or speak at meetings or local groups. By doing so you may be able to get a feel for the kind of person he or she is and his or her ability to help you.

6. *Look for a person who is open-minded,* up-to-date, and willing to try new things.

7. *Look for a person who treats you with respect,* listens to your questions, and responds to your needs. Look for a relationship that is collaborative and respectful.

We know it is hard to find a professional who meets all of these criteria and who also has the right training in brain physiology, but these people can be found. Be persistent. The professional is essential to healing.

The national Alzheimer's Association is a very good referral source. They have hundreds of local chapters and can often refer you to a local specialist.

Frequently Asked Questions About Brain SPECT Imaging

❀ *Will the SPECT study give me an accurate diagnosis?* No. A SPECT study by itself will not give a diagnosis. The SPECT studies help the clinician understand more about the specific function of your brain. Each person's brain is unique, and this may lead to unique responses to medicine or therapy. Diagnoses about specific conditions are made through a combination of clinical history, personal interview, information from families, diagnostic checklists, SPECT studies, and other neuropsychological tests. No study is "a doctor in a box" that can give accurate diagnoses on an individual patient.

Why are SPECT studies ordered? Some of the common reasons include:

1. Evaluating memory problems and dementia and distinguishing between different types of dementia and pseudodementia (depression that looks like dementia)
2. Evaluating seizure activity
3. Evaluating blood vessel diseases, such as stroke
4. Evaluating the effects of mild, moderate, and severe head trauma
5. Suspicion of underlying organic brain condition, such as seizure activity contributing to behavioral disturbance, prenatal trauma, or exposure to toxins
6. Evaluating atypical or unresponsive aggressive behavior
7. Determining the extent of brain impairment caused by drug or alcohol abuse
8. Typing anxiety, depression, and attention deficit disorders when clinical presentation is not clear

Do I need to be off medication before the study? This question must be answered individually by you and your doctor. In general, it is better to be off medications until they are out of your system, but this is not always practical or advisable. If the study is done while on medication, let the technician know, so that when the physician reads the study he or she will include that information in the interpretation of the scan. In general, we recommend that patients try to be off stimulants at least four days before the first scan and remain off them until after the second scan if one is ordered. It is generally not practical to stop medications such as Prozac, because they last in the body for four to six weeks. Check with your specific doctor for recommendations.

What should I do the day of the scan? Decrease or eliminate your caffeine intake and try to avoid taking cold medication or aspirin (if you do, please write it down on the intake form). Eat as you normally would.

Are there any side effects or risks to the study? The study does not involve a dye, and people do not have allergic reactions to the study. The possibility exists, although in a very small percentage of patients, of a mild rash, facial redness and edema, fever, and a transient increase in blood pressure. The amount of radiation exposure from one brain SPECT study is approximately the same as one abdominal X-ray.

How is the SPECT procedure done? The patient is placed in a quiet room, and a small intravenous (IV) line is started. The patient remains quiet for approximately 10 minutes with his or her eyes open to allow the mental state to equilibrate to the environment. The imaging agent is then injected through the IV. After another short period of time, the patient lies on a table, and the SPECT camera rotates around his or her head (the patient does not go into a tube). The time on the table is approximately 15 minutes. If a concentration study is ordered, the patient returns on another day.

Are there alternatives to having a SPECT study? In our opinion, SPECT is the most clinically useful study of brain function. There are other studies, such as electroencephalographs (EEGs), positron emission tomography (PET) studies, and functional MRIs (fMRI). PET studies and fMRIs are considerably more costly, and they are performed mostly in research settings. EEGs, in our opinion, do not provide enough information about the deep structures of the brain to be as helpful as SPECT studies.

Does insurance cover the cost of SPECT studies? Reimbursement by insurance companies varies according to your plan. It is often a good idea to check with the insurance company ahead of time to see if it is a covered benefit.

Is the use of brain SPECT imaging accepted in the medical community? Yes; brain SPECT studies are widely recognized as an effective tool for evaluating brain function in seizures, strokes, dementia, and head trauma. There are literally hundreds of research articles on these topics. In our clinic, on the basis of our experience for over a decade, we have developed this technology further to evaluate aggression and nonresponsive psychiatric conditions. Unfortunately, many physicians do not fully understand the application of SPECT imaging and may tell you that the technology is experimental, but over 350 physicians in the United States have referred patients to us for scans.

References

1. Shankle R, Rafii MS, Landing BH. Functional relationships associated with pattern of developing in developing human cerebral cortex. *Concepts in Neuroscience* 4, 1: 77–87, 1993.
2. Shankle WR, Landing BH, Rafii MS, Schiano AVR, Chen JM, Hara J. Numbers of neurons per column in the developing human cerebral cortex from birth to 72 months: Evidence for an apparent post-natal increase in neuron numbers. *J Theor Biol* 191: 115–40, 1998.
3. Erikkson PS, Bjork-Eriksson T, Alborn AM, Nordborg C, Peterson DA, Gage FH, Perfilieva E. Neurogenesis in the adult human hippocampus. *Nat Med* 4: 1313–7, 1998.
4. Sano M. A controlled trial of selegiline, alpha-tocopherol, or both as treatment for Alzheimer's disease. *New Eng J Med* 336: 1216–22, 1997.

5. Engelhart MJ, Geerlings MI, Ruitenberg A, van Swieten JC, Hofman, A, Witteman JC, Breteler MM. Dietary intake of antioxidants and risk of Alzheimer's disease. *JAMA* 287: 3261–3, 2002.

6. Le Bars PL, Katz MM, Berman N, Itil TM, Freedman AM, Schatzberg AF. A placebo-controlled, double-blind, randomized trial of an extract of Ginkgo biloba for dementia. North American EGb Study Group. *JAMA* 278: 1327–32, 1997.

7. Van Dongen MC, van Rossum E, Kessels AG, Sielhorst HJ, Knipschild PG. The efficacy of ginkgo for elderly people with dementia and age-associated memory impairment: New results of a randomized clinical trial. *J Am Geriatr Soc* 48: 1183–94, 2000.

8. Hager K. Marahrens A, Kenklies M, Riederer P, Munch G. Alphalipoic acid as a new treatment option for Alzheimer type dementia. *Arch Gerontol Geriatr* 32: 275–82, 2001.

9. Reisberg B, Doody R, Stoffler A, Ferris S, Mobius HJ. Memantine in moderate-to-severe Alzheimer's disease. Memantine Study Group. *N Engl J Med* 348: 1333–41, 2003.

10. Auriacombe S, Pere JJ, Loria-Kanza Y, Vellas B. Efficacy and safety of rivastigmine in patients with Alzheimer's disease who failed to benefit from treatment with donepezil. *Curr Med Res Opin* 18: 129–38, 2002.

11. Andersen K, Ott A, Hoes AW, Launer LJ, Breiteler MB, Hofman A. Do nonsteroidal anti-inflammatory drugs decrease the risk of Alzheimer's disease? *Neurology* 45: 1441–5, 1995.

12. Breitner JC, Gau BA, Welsh KA. Inverse association of antiinflammatory treatments and Alzheimer's disease: Initial results of a co-twin control study. *Neurology* 44: 227–32, 1994.

13. Stewart WF. Risk of Alzheimer's disease and duration of NSAID use. *Neurology* 48: 626–32, 1997.

14. McGeer PL, McGeer E, Rogers J. Anti-inflammatory drugs and Alzheimer's disease. *Lancet* 335: 1037, 1990.

15. Bernhardt T, Maurer K, Frolich L. Effect of daily living-related cognitive training on attention and memory performance of persons with dementia. *Z Gerontol Geriatr* 35: 32–8, 2002.

16. Clare L, Wilson BA, Carter G, Roth I, Hodges JR. Relearning face-

name associations in early Alzheimer's disease. *Neuropsychology* 16: 538–47, 2002.

17. Bergsneider M, Hovda DA, McArthur DL, Etchepare M, Huang SC, Sehati N, Satz P, Phelps ME, Becker DP. Metabolic recovery following human traumatic brain injury based on FDG-PET: Time course and relationship to neurological disability. *J Head Trauma Rehabil* 16: 135–48, 2001.

18. Laurin D, Verreault R, Lindsay J, MacPherson K, Rockwood K. Physical activity and risk of cognitive impairment and dementia in elderly persons. *Arch Neurol* 58: 498–504, 2001.

19. Rozzini R, Ferrucci L, Losonczy K, Havlik RJ, Guralnik JM. Protective effect of chronic NSAID use on cognitive decline in older persons. *J Am Geriatr Soc* 44: 1025–9, 1996.

20. Ma Q, Wang J, Liu HT, Chao FH. [Attentuation of chronic stress-induced hippocampal damages following physical exercise]. *Sheng Li Xue Bao* 54: 427–30, 2002.

21. Murialdo G, Barreca A, Nobili F, Rollero A, Timossi G, Gianelli MV, Copello F, Rodriguez G, Polleri A. Relationships between cortisol, dehydroepiandrosterone sulphate and insulin-like growth factor-I system in dementia. *J Endocrinol Invest* 24: 139–46, 2001.

22. Launer LJ, Masaki K, Petrovitch H, Foley D, Havlik RJ. The association between midlife blood pressure levels and late-life cognitive function. The Honolulu-Asia Aging Study. *JAMA* 274: 1846–51, 1995.

23. Cotman CW, Berchtold NC. Exercise: a behavioral intervention to enhance brain health and plasticity. *Trends Neurosci* 25: 295–301, 2002.

24. Broe GA, Creasey H, Jorm AF, Bennett HP, Casey B, Waite LM, Grayson DA, Cullen J. Health habits and risk of cognitive impairment and dementia in old age: A prospective study on the effects of exercise, smoking and alcohol consumption. *Aust N Z J Public Health* 22: 621–3, 1998.

25. Wilson RS, Bienias JL, Berry-Kravis E, Evans DA, Bennett DA. The apolipoprotein E varepsilon 2 allele and decline in episodic memory. *J Neurol Neurosurg Psychiatry* 73: 672–7, 2002.

26. Braak H, Braak E. Evolution of the neuropathology of Alzheimer's disease. *Acta Neurol Scand Suppl* 165: 3–12, 1996.

27. Fillit H. Treating Alzheimer's disease and the economic impact on managed care. *Clinical Geriatrics* 10–3, 2001.

28. Landing BH, Shankle WR. Considerations of quantitative data on organ sizes and cell numbers and sizes in Down syndrome. *Progress in Clinical and Biological Research* 393: 177–91, 1995.

29. Hansen LAea. Neocortical morphometry, lesion counts, and choline acetyltransferase levels in the age spectrum of Alzheimer's disease. *Neurology* 38: 48–54, 1988.

30. Braak E, Griffing K, Arai K, Bohl J, Bratzke H, Braak H. Neuropathology of Alzheimer's disease: What is new since A. Alzheimer? *Eur Arch Psychiatry Clin Neurosci* 249 Suppl 3: 14–22, 1999.

31. *Consensus panel. Vascular dementia: The basics with case presentations.* National Stroke Association, 2002.

32. Tang MX, Maestre G, Tsai WY, Liu XH, Feng L, Chung WY, Chun M, Schofield P, Stern Y, Tycko B, Mayeux R. Effect of age, ethnicity, and head injury on the association between APOE genotypes and Alzheimer's disease. *Ann N Y Acad Sci* 802: 6–15, 1996.

33. Truelson T. Amount and type of alcohol and risk of dementia: The Copenhagen City Heart Study. *Neurology* 59: 1313–9, 2002.

34. Nagy Z, Hindley NJ, Braak H, Braak E, Yilmazer-Hanke DM, Schultz C, Barnetson L, Jobst KA, Smith AD. Relationship between clinical and radiological diagnostic criteria for Alzheimer's disease and the extent of neuropathology as reflected by "stages": A prospective study. *Dement Geriatr Cogn Disord* 10: 109–14, 1999.

35. Ibid.

36. Corbo RM, Scacchi R. Apolipoprotein E (APOE) allele distribution in the world. Is APOE4 a "thrifty" allele? *Ann Hum Genet* 63: 301–10, 1999.

37. Bird TD. Clinical genetics of familial Alzheimer Disease. In: Terry RD, Katzman R, Bick KL, Sisson RA, eds. *Alzheimer Disease*. Philadelphia: Lippincott Williams & Wilkins, 57–67, 1999.

38. Selkoe DJ. AD: genotypes, phenotype and treatment. *Science* 275: 630–1, 1997.

39. Papadakis JA, Ganotakis ES, Mikhailidis DP. Beneficial effect of moderate alcohol consumption on vascular disease: Myth or reality? *J R Soc Health* 120: 11–5, 2000.

40. Van Dam FS, Schagen SB, Muller MJ, Boogerd W, van de Wall E, Droogleever Fortuyn ME, Rodenhuis S. Impairment of cognitive function in women receiving adjuvant treatment for high-risk breast cancer: High-dose versus standard-dose chemotherapy. *J Natl Cancer Inst* 90: 210–8, 1998.

41. Kosunen O, Talasniemi S, Lehtovirta M, Heinonen O, Helisalmi S, Mannermaa A, Paljarvi L, Ryynanen M, Riekkinen PJ, Sr., Soininen H. Relation of coronary atherosclerosis and apolipoprotein E genotypes in Alzheimer patients. *Stroke* 26: 743–8, 1995.

42. Rockwood K, Kirkland S, Hogan DB, MacKnight C, Merry H, Verreault R, Wolfson C, McDowell I. Use of lipid-lowering agents, indication bias, and the risk of dementia in community-dwelling elderly people. *Arch Neurol* 59: 223–7, 2002.

43. Van Kooten F, Bots ML, Breteler MM, Haverkate F, van Swieten JC, Grobbee DE, Koudstaal PJ, Kluft C. The Dutch Vascular Factors in Dementia Study: Rationale and design. *J Neurol* 245: 32–9, 1998.

44. Yaffe K, Lui LY, Grady D, Stone K, Morin P. Estrogen receptor 1 polymorphisms and risk of cognitive impairment in older women. *Biol Psychiatry* 51: 677–82, 2002.

45. Kalmijn S, Foley D, White L, Burchfiel CM, Curb JD, Petrovitch H, Ross GW, Havlik RJ, Launer LJ. Metabolic cardiovascular syndrome and risk of dementia in Japanese-American elderly men. The Honolulu-Asia Aging Study. *Arterioscler Thromb Vasc Biol* 20: 2255–60, 2000.

46. Menku A, Koc RK, Tayfur V, Saraymen R, Narin F, Akdemir H. Effects of mexiletine, ginkgo biloba extyract (EGb 761), and their combination on experimental head injury. *Neurosurg Rev* 2003.

47. Weggen S, Eriksen JL, Das P, Sagi SA, Wang R, Pietrzik CU, Findlay KA, Smith TE, Murphy MP, Bulter T, Kang DE, Marquez-Sterling N, Golde TE, Koo EH. A subset of NSAIDs lower amyloidogenic Abeta42 independently of cyclooxygenase activity. *Nature* 414: 212–6, 2001.

48. Jacobs B, Schall M, Scheibel AB. A quantitative dendritic analysis of

Wernicke's area in humans. II. Gender, hemispheric, and environmental factors. *J Comp Neurol* 327: 97–111, 1993.

49. Seshadri S, Beiser A, Selhub J, Jacques PF, Rosenberg IH, D'Agostino RB, Wilson PW, Wolf PA. Plasma homocysteine as a risk factor for dementia and Alzheimer's disease. *N Engl J Med* 346: 476–83, 2002.

50. Schnyder G, Roffi M, Pin R, Flammer Y, Lange H, Eberli FR, Meier B, Turi ZG, Hess OM. Decreased rate of coronary restenosis after lowering of plasma homocysteine levels. *N Engl J Med* 345: 1593–1600, 2001.

51. Kawas C, Resnick S, Morrison A, Brookmeyer R, Corrada M, Zonderman A, Bacal C, Lingle DD, Metter E. A prospective study of estrogen replacement therapy and the risk of developing Alzheimer's disease: The Baltimore Longitudinal Study of Aging. *Neurology* 48: 1517–21, 1997.

52. McCleary R, Mulnard RA, Shankle WR. Reproductive health risks in dementia: Evidence from the 1986 National Mortality Followback Survey. *Alzheimer's Research* 2: 181–4, 1996.

53. Ficker JH, Feistel H, Moller C, Merkl M, Dertinger S, Siegfried W, Hahn EG. [Changes in regional CNS perfusion in obstructive sleep apnea syndrome: Initial SPECT studies with injected nocturnal 99mTc-HMPAO]. *Pneumologie* 51: 926–30, 1997.

54. Brooks JO, Yesavage JA, Carta A, Bravi D. Acetyl L-carnitine slows decline in younger patients with Alzheimer's disease: A reanalysis of a double-blind, placebo-controlled study using the trilinear approach. *Int Psychogeriatr* 10: 193–203, 1998.

55. Di Castelnuovo A, Rotondo S, Iacoviello L, Donati MB, De Gaetano G. Meta-analysis of wine and beer consumption in relation to vascular risk. *Circulation* 105: 2836–44, 2002.

56. Ruitenberg A, van Swieten JC, Witteman JC, Mehta KM, van Duijn CM, Hofman A, Breteler MM. Alcohol consumption and risk of dementia: The Rotterdam Study. *Lancet* 359: 281–6, 2002.

57. Zhang L, Xing GQ, Barker JL, Chang Y, Maric D, Ma W, Li BS, Rubinow DR. Alpha-lipoic acid protects rat coritcal neurons against cell death induced by amyloid and hydrogen peroxide through the Akt signalling pathway. *Neurosci Lett* 312: 125–8, 2001.

58. Clark WM, Rinker LG, Lessov NS, Lowery SL, Cipolla MJ. Efficacy of antioxidant therapies in transient focal ischemia in mice. *Stroke* 32: 1000–4, 2001.

59. Kawas C, Katzman R. Epidemiolotgy of dementia and Alzheimer's disease. In: Terry RD, Katzman R, Bick KL, Sisson RA, eds. *Alzheimer Disease.* Philadelphia: Lippincott Williams & Wilkins, 95–117, 1999.

60. Shults CW, Oakes D, Kieburtz K, Beal MF, Haas R, Plumb S, Juncos JL, Nutt J, Shoulson I, Carter J, Kompoliti K, Perlmutter JS, Reich S, Stern M, Watts RL, Kurlan R, Molho E, Harrison M, Lew M. Effects of coenzyme Q10 in early Parkinson disease: Evidence of slowing of the functional decline. *Arch Neurol* 59: 1541–50, 2002.

61. Luchsinger JA, Tang MX, Shea S, Mayeux R. Caloric intake and the risk of Alzheimer's disease. *Arch Neurol* 59: 1258–63, 2002.

62. Conquer JA, Tierney MC, Zecevic J, Bettger WJ, Fisher RH. Fatty acid analysis of blood plasma of patients with Alzheimer's disease, other types of dementia, and cognitive impairment. *Lipids* 35: 1305–12, 2000.

63. Morris MC, Evans DA, Bienias JL, Tangney CC, Wilson RS. Vitamin E and cognitive decline in older persons. *Arch Neurol* 59: 1125–32, 2002.

64. Sweeney MI, Kalt W, MacKinnon SL, Ashby J, Gottschall-Pass KT. Feeding rats diets enriched in lowbush blueberries for six weeks decreases ischemia-induced brain damage. *Nutr Neurosci* 5: 427–31, 2002.

65. Nelson HD, Humphrey LL, Nygren P, Teutsch SM, Allan JD. Postmenopausal hormone replacement therapy: Scientific review. *JAMA* 288: 872–81, 2002.

66. Farrag AK, Khedr EM. Effect of surgical menopause on cognitive functions. *Dement Geriatr Cogn Disord* 13: 193–8, 2002.

67. Kabuto M, Akiba S, Stevens RG, Neriishi K, Land CE. A prospective study of estradiol and breast cancer in Japanese women. *Cancer Epidemiol Biomarkers Prev* 9: 575–9, 2000.

68. Wettstein A. Cholinesterase inhibitors and Ginkgo extracts—are they comparable in the treatment of dementia? Comparison of published placebo-controlled efficacy studies of at least six months' duration. *Phytomedicine* 6: 393–401, 2000.

69. Sasaki Y, Noguchi T, Yamamoto E, Giddings JC, Ikeda K, Yamori Y, Yamamoto J. Effects of Ginkgo biloba extract (EGb 761) on cerebral thrombosis and blood pressure in stroke-prone spontaneously hypertensive rats. *Clin Exp Pharmacol Physiol* 29: 963–7, 2002.

70. Wilson RS, Mendes De Leon CF, Barnes LL, Schneider JA, Bienias JL, Evans DA, Bennett DA. Participation in cognitively stimulating activities and risk of incident Alzheimer disease. *JAMA* 287: 742–8, 2002.

71. Jantzen PT, Connor KE, DiCarlo G, Wenk GL, Wallace JL, Rojiani AM, Coppola D, Morgan D, Gordon MN. Microglial activation and beta-amyloid deposit reduction caused by a nitric oxide-releasing nonsteroidal anti-inflammatory drug in amyloid precursor protein plus presenilin-1 transgenic mice. *J Neurosci* 22: 2246–54, 2002.

72. Newton AC, Keranen LM. Phosphatidyl-L-serine is necessary for protein kinase C's high-affinity interaction with diacylglycerol-containing membranes. *Biochemistry* 33: 6651–8, 1994.

73. Heiss WD, Szelies B, Kessler J, Herholz K. Abnormalities of energy metabolism in Alzheimer's disease studied with PET. *Ann N Y Acad Sci* 640: 65–71, 1991.

74. Rimm EB, Willett WC, Hu FB, Sampson L, Colditz GA, Manson JE, Hennekens C, Stampfer MJ. Folate and vitamin B6 from diet and supplements in relation to risk of coronary heart disease among women. *JAMA* 279: 359–64, 1998.

75. Valcour VG, Masaki KH, Curb JD, Blanchette PL. The detection of dementia in the primary care setting. *Arch Intern Med* 160: 2964–8, 2000.

76. Gifford DR, Cummings JL. Rating dementia screening tests: methodologic standards to rate their performance. *Neurology* 52: 224–7, 1999.

77. Darreh-Shori T, Almkvist O, Guan ZZ, Garlind A, Strandberg B, Svensson Al, Soreq H, Hellstrom-Lindahl E, Nordberg A. Sustained cholinesterase inhibition in AD patients receiving rivastigmine for 12 months. *Neurology* 59: 563–72, 2002.

78. Santos MD, Alkondon M, Pereira EF, Aracava Y, Eisenberg HM, Maelick A, Albuquerque EX. The nicotinic allosteric potentiating ligand galantamine facilitates synaptic transmission in the mammalian central nervous system. *Mol Pharmacol* 61: 1222–34, 2004.

79. Goldsmith HS. *The Omentum: Application to Brain and Spinal Cord.* Wilton, CT: Forefront, 2000.

80. Bikfalvi A, Alterio J. Basic fibroblast growth factor expression in human omental microvascular endothelial cells and the effect of phorbol ester. *J Cellular Physiol* 144: 151–8, 1990.

81. Siek GC, Marquis JK. Experimental studies of omentum-derived neurotrophic factors. In: H. S. Goldsmith, ed. *The Omentum: Research and Clinical Applications.* New York: Springer-Verlag, 1990, pp. 83–95.

82. Goldsmith HS, Marquis JK. Choline acetyltransferase activity in omental tissue. *Br J Neurosurg* 1: 463–6, 1987.

83. Relkin NR, Edgar MA, Gouras GK, Gandy SE, Goldsmith HS. Decreased senile plaque density in Alzheimer neocortex adjacent to an omental transposition. *Neurol Res* 18: 291–6, 1996.

84. Zhang QX, Magovern CJ. Vascular endothelial growth factor is the major angiogenic factor in omentum: Mechanism for the omentum-mediated angiogenesis. *J Surg Res* 67: 147–54, 1997.

85. Frey WH. Intranasal delivery: Bypassing the blood-brain barrier to deliver therapeutic agents to the brain and spinal cord. *Drug Delivery Technology* 2: 46–9, 2002.

86. Jin K, Xie L, Childs J, Sun Y, Mao XO, Logvinova A, Greenberg DA. Cerebral neurogenesis is induced by intranasal administration of growth factors. *Ann Neurol* 53: 405–9, 2003.

87. Miller III ER, Pastor-Barriuso R, Dalal D, Riemersma RA, Appel LJ, Guallar E. Meta-Analysis: High-dose Vitamin E supplementation may increase all-cause mortality. *Annals of Internal Medicine* 142 (1), 2004.

Glossary

acetylcholine (ACh) A neurotransmitter involved with memory formation, mostly excitatory; has been implicated in problems with muscles, Alzheimer's disease, and learning problems.

acetyl-L-carnitine (ALC) An amino acid involved in the transport of fatty acids into the cell's mitochondria for the purpose of producing energy. May be helpful in preventing strokes and heart attacks.

action potential Electrical signal generated by neurons.

adenosine triphosphate (ATP) Energy molecule within cells.

atrial fibrillation A fluttering (arrhythmia) of the heart that reduces the amount of blood it can pump.

alpha lipoic acid (ALA) Powerful antioxidant that increases the potency of many other antioxidants.

alpha-synuclein gene On chromosome 4; involved with producing the most common form of Parkinson's disease.

Alzheimer's disease (AD) Most common form of dementia; results from beta amyloid production and neurofibrillary tangles.

Alzheimer's disease and related disorders (ADRD) A group of disorders that includes Alzheimer's disease, vascular dementia, frontal-temporal lobe dementia, Lewy body disease, and other common causes of dementia.

amyloid precursor protein (APP) A normal protein necessary for brain development and repair. After it is used, APP gets broken down into a harmless 37-amino-acid fragment, which is then recycled back into APP; sometimes it is broken down in beta amyloid, which is believed to be a major cause of Alzheimer's disease.

antioxidants Substances that help to prevent damage from free-radical formation.

apolipoprotein E (apoE) gene Gene involved in the development, maturation, and repair of cell membranes of neurons; also helps regulate the amount of cholesterol and triglycerides in nerve cell membranes. There are three versions of the apoE gene: E2, E3, and E4, and it is the last one that increases the risk for Alzheimer's disease, as well as a number of other illnesses.

atherosclerosis Hardening of the arteries from excessive fatty plaque deposition.

axon Usually a long nerve fiber that projects from the cell body to connect with other cells.

beta amyloid (BA42) Protein breakdown product that combines with salt and water to form the toxic neuritic plaques of Alzheimer's disease.

beta amyloid plaques Conglomeration of toxic material including beta amyloid protein, which disrupts normal nerve transmission.

beta secretase An enzyme that breaks down amyloid precursor protein into a 40- or 42-amino-acid fragment, both of which are called beta amyloid. The 42-amino-acid fragment (BA42) is believed to be a major cause of Alzheimer's disease.

brain-derived neurotrophic factor (BDNF) Experimental nerve growth factor used to treat AD.

carotid bruit Narrowing of blood vessel in the neck.

cat's claw *(Uncaria tomentosa)* Plant found in South America, the inner bark of which contains compounds that in test tubes block the formation of the toxic form of beta amyloid. Not yet known if helpful in humans.

central nervous system (CNS) The system that is composed of the spinal cord and parts of the brain, brain stem, thalamus, basal ganglia, cerebellum, and cerebral cortex.

cerebrolysin (Cere) Drug that encourages nerve growth factor.

cholinergic neurons Neurons that produce the neurotransmitter acetylcholine.

chronic fatigue immunodeficiency syndrome (CFIDS) A combination of immune deficiency plus infection by any of a number of infectious agents that are normally destroyed by the immune system. Often associated with cognitive impairment, lethargy, and depression.

Coenzyme Q10 (CoQ10) Enzyme that lives inside the battery of your cells (the mitochondria) and helps convert oxygen into usable cellular energy, called ATP.

COGNIShunt Trade name of a low-flow shunt currently under investigation as a possible treatment for dementia.

Creutzfeld-Jakob disease (CJD) or **"mad cow disease"** A rare form of dementia caused by an infectious agent called a prion, which can be transmitted by farm animals such as cows or sheep, by infected people undergoing neurosurgery or corneal transplants, or by an infected person who has donated a pituitary gland for growth hormones.

dendrites Structures that branch out from the cell body and serve as the main receivers of signals from other nerve cells and function as the "antennae" of the neuron.

dopamine (DA) A neurotransmitter involved with attention, motor movements, and motivation; has been implicated in Parkinson's disease, attention deficit disorder, addictions, depression, and schizophrenia.

Down syndrome Congenital disorder associated with an extra copy of chromosome 21; associated with typical facial features, mental retardation, and early-onset Alzheimer's disease.

Entorhinal cortex An important transitional part of the brain on the inside of the temporal lobes that packages what you want to learn and sends it to the hippocampus for encoding into memory.

evidence-based medicine (EBM) A process that involves asking clear questions of the published scientific literature to ascertain how much claims and results should be trusted.

EBM level 1: *group studies* Highest reliability

EBM level 2: *case-control studies* Second-highest reliability

EBM level 3: *case series studies* Third-highest reliability

EBM level 4: *animal studies* Fourth-highest reliability

EBM level 5: *test tube or tissue research* Lowest reliability

fMRI A brain scan that uses powerful magnets to look at brain blood flow and activity patterns.

free radicals Oxygen combines with other molecules to generate these highly toxic substances; they must be neutralized by antioxidants or they cause damage to cells.

frontal-temporal lobe dementia (FTLD) A type of dementia characterized by deterioration of the frontal and temporal lobes, associated with apathy, poor judgment, and memory problems.

gamma-aminobutyric acid (GABA) An inhibitory neurotransmitter involved with calming brain function; has been implicated in problems with seizures, bipolar disorder, anxiety, and pain.

gamma secretase Enzyme that breaks down amyloid precursor protein into a 40- or 42-amino-acid fragment, both of which are called beta amyloid. The 42-amino-acid fragment (BA42) is believed to be a major cause of Alzheimer's disease.

ginkgo biloba Herb from the Chinese ginkgo tree that is known to improve circulation and blood flow and has been shown to be helpful in dementia.

glutamate Excitatory (stimulating) neurotransmitter.

glutamate receptor modifiers (mGluRs) Drugs that have the protective effects of certain glutamate receptors against the overproduction of glutamate, which is toxic to the brain.

hippocampus Part of the inside of the temporal lobes that facilitates memory function.

homocysteine Amino acid that when elevated increases the risk for AD.

hyperlipidemia High total or LDL cholesterol.

lacunar infarcts Small strokes.

leteprinim (Neotrofin) Drug that activates genes that produce nerve growth factor.

Lewy body disease (LBD) A common form of dementia caused by the deposition of an abnormal substance called Lewy bodies; often associated with Parkinson's disease.

locus ceruleus (LC) Clusters of cells in the brain stem that produce the neurotransmitter norepinephrine.

long-term potentiation (LTP) The process of invigorating (or potentiating) neurons to do their job over a long period of time; it is accomplished through the repetition of an act, which causes actual physical changes in neurons and their synapses.

low-flow shunts Devices that drain cerebrospinal fluid from the brain; may be helpful in AD.

magnetic resonance imaging (MRI) A type of brain scan that uses powerful magnets to look at the physical structure of organs.

melatonin Naturally produced hormone that helps regulate sleep-wake cycles.

memantine (Namenda) An NMDA antagonist; a drug that may have the protective effects of certain glutamate receptors against the overproduction of glutamate, which is toxic in large amounts.

myelin The whitish fatty substance rich in proteins and lipids that covers neurons.

myelination The act of laying down myelin onto neurons.

nerve growth factor (NGF) One of several growth factors in the brain that promote the regeneration of nerve cells after injury.

neurofibrillary tangles (NFT) Mutations of a gene on chromosome 17 have been found to cause the tau protein (backbone of nerve cells) to twist into a spiral staircase, blocking the flow of molecules from the cell body to the outer regions and causing the cell to wither and die.

neurogenesis The growth of new neurons.

neuron Synonymous with *nerve cell.*

neurotransmitter A chemical that is released from one neuron at the pre-synaptic nerve terminal (the end of an axon) and crosses the synapse, where it may be accepted by the next neuron (on the dendrites) at a specialized site called a receptor. There are many different neuro-transmitters, such as acetylcholine, serotonin, dopamine, and norepinephrine.

neurotrophin-3 Experimental nerve growth factor used to treat AD.

N-methyl D-aspartate (NMDA) A type of glutamate receptor known for its ability to cause nerve cell death.

Nonsteroidal anti-inflammatory medications (NSAIDs) Common painkilling medications that work in part by decreasing inflammation and thinning the blood. Some NSAIDs also appear to block the production of beta amyloid.

norepinephrine (NE) A neurotransmitter involved with mood, concentration, and motivation and thought be associated with problems of attention, depression, and anxiety.

normal-pressure hydrocephalus An illness, caused by an increase in the production of cerebral spinal fluid, that results in early symptoms of difficulty walking, urinary incontinence, and cognitive impairment.

omental transposition surgery (OTS) A surgery that involves placing the abdominal structure known as the omentum directly onto the brain. It has been reported to be helpful in a number of Alzheimer's disease patients and was pioneered by the surgeon Harry Goldsmith.

Parkinson's disease (PD) Caused by loss of neurons that produce the neurotransmitter dopamine in a part of the brain stem called the substantia nigra, often associated with a tremor, slowed movements, and rigidity; PD is often associated with dementia after three years.

peripheral nervous system (PNS) The system composed of receptors in the internal organs (outside the brain) and in skin, muscle tendons, eyes, ears, nose, and tongue.

positron emission tomography (PET) A type of brain scan that uses isotopes to look at glucose metabolism and activity patterns in the brain.

postsynaptic membrane The receiving end of a dendrite that has receptors that are signaled by neurotransmitters released from the presynaptic terminals of axons.

presenilin 1 gene (PS1) Gene mutation on chromosome 14 that greatly accelerates beta amyloid production; causes Alzheimer's disease symptoms to appear when people are between 35 and 65 years old.

presenilin 2 gene (PS2) Gene mutation on chromosome 1 that greatly accelerates beta amyloid production. More rare than PS1; causes Alzheimer's disease symptoms to appear between ages 40 and 85.

presynaptic membrane The terminal end of the axon, where neurotransmitters are released.

serotonin (5-HT) A neurotransmitter involved with mood, flexibility, shifting attention; often involved with problems of depression, obsessive compulsive disorder, eating disorders, sleep disturbances, pain.

single photon emission computed tomography (SPECT) A type of brain scan that uses isotopes to look at blood flow and activity patterns in the brain.

statins Drugs to lower cholesterol.

stem cells Basic or primordial cells from which all human tissues and organs develop; they have the potential to differentiate, or specialize, into each of the two hundred types of tissue in the body, such as heart cells, bone cells, cartilage cells, liver cells, and even brain cells.

substantia nigra A part of the basal ganglia in the brain stem that produces the neurotransmitter dopamine; deficits here are known to be involved in Parkinson's disease.

synapses Junctions formed between nerve cells where the presynaptic terminal of an axon comes into "contact" with the dendrite's postsynaptic membrane of another neuron. There are two types of synapses: electrical and chemical.

synaptic plasticity The ability of synapses to change to more efficiently signal other neurons.

tau protein Protein that normally forms the neuron's basic shape and backbone. Tau proteins look like steel girders that give the neurons its characteristic shape, which can be anything from a star to a pyramid. Abnormalities of the tau protein have been implicated in Alzheimer's disease, causing neurofibrillary tangles that block healthy cell function.

transforming growth factor alpha (TGF-alpha) A nerve growth factor that encourages the proliferation of stem cells.

transient ischemic attack (TIA) Temporary stroke that reverses itself within 24 hours.

use-dependent plasticity "Use it or lose it": neurons or their connections that are not periodically activated wither away from disuse.

vascular dementia (VD) A common cause of dementia associated with problems in circulation of blood to the brain.

vinpocetine Derived from an extract of the common periwinkle plant (*Vinca minor*); it is a cerebral vasodilator, increasing blood flow to the brain, and may be helpful for Alzheimer's disease, vascular dementia, and cardiovascular illnesses.

Resources

Medical Care Corporation: Prevention Through Delay

Medical Care Corporation (MCC) develops knowledge-ware specialized for the prevention, early detection, accurate diagnosis, and effective treatment of dementia due to Alzheimer's Disease and Related Disorders (ADRD).

MCC has successfully used advanced mathematical algorithms to improve the ability to detect ADRD in its earliest and most treatable stages. Coupled with MCC's suite of electronic knowledge-ware for physicians, this breakthrough has greatly improved treatment outcomes for Alzheimer's disease and has given the public the opportunity to prevent Alzheimer's disease by delaying its onset and progression beyond the expected life of the individual. MCC calls this concept Prevention Through Delay.

The website sponsored by MCC, www.PreventAD.com, is for readers like yourself who are interested in prevention, early detection, and treatment of ADRD so that it does not ruin the lives of you and your family. This website offers public access to MCC's powerful screening and prevention tools, which currently include the Memory Screen, the Depression Screen, and the Mental Skills Test. The website also provides useful information about ADRD, as well as information to help caregivers and families affected by ADRD. Since it is now well established that the key to effective treatment is early detection, the Memory Screen and Mental Skills Test provide the public and medical professionals with the opportunity to detect the earliest signs of mental decline with 98 percent accuracy, and dramatically improve the lives of affected individuals and their loved ones.

Medical Care Corporation
19782 MacArthur Blvd., Suite 310
Irvine, CA 92612
www.mccare.com

The Shankle Clinic

Established in 1997, the Shankle Clinic grew out of the 10 years of experience Dr. Shankle gathered in treating ADRD patients and their families at the Alzheimer's Disease Research Center at the University of California, Irvine, where he served as its medical director. During that time he received numerous grants to develop better ways to improve the evaluation and treatment of ADRD.

Dr. Shankle has evaluated, treated, and managed thousands of ADRD patients during his career, which is solely devoted to the assessment of cognitive impairment, behavioral problems, and dementia due to ADRD.

The Shankle Clinic specializes in screening for early-stage ADRD and the diagnosis, treatment, monitoring, and management of ADRD. It also provides education and counseling for patients, caregivers, and their families, as well as prevention planning and risk management for ADRD.

The Shankle Clinic
19782 MacArthur Blvd., Suite 310
Irvine, CA 92612
949-833-2383
www.ShankleClinic.com

Amen Clinics, Inc.

The Amen Clinics were established in 1989 by Daniel G. Amen, M.D. They specialize in innovative diagnosis and treatment planning for a wide variety of behavioral, learning, and emotional problems for children, teenagers, and adults. The clinics have an international reputation for evaluating brain-behavior problems such as attention deficit disorder (ADD), depression, anxiety, school failure, brain trauma, obsessive-compulsive disorders, aggressiveness, cognitive decline, and brain toxicity from drugs or alcohol. Brain SPECT imaging is performed in the clinics. Amen Clinics have the world's largest database of brain scans for behavioral problems. Over the last twelve years, they have performed over 20,000 brain SPECT studies.

The clinics welcome referrals from physicians, psychologists, social workers, marriage and family therapists, drug and alcohol counselors, and individual clients.

Amen Clinics, Inc., Newport Beach
4019 Westerly Place, Suite 100
Newport Beach, CA 92660
(949) 266-3700

Amen Clinics, Inc., Fairfield
350 Chadbourne Road
Fairfield, CA 94585
(707) 429-7181

Amen Clinics, Inc., Northwest
3315 South 23rd Street

Tacoma, WA
(253) 779-HOPE

Amen Clinics, Inc., D.C.
1875 Campus Commons Drive
Suite 101
Reston, VA 20191
(703) 860-5600
website: www.amenclinic.com

Brainplace.com

Brainplace.com is an educational interactive brain website geared toward mental health and medical professionals, educators, students, and the general public. It contains a wealth of information to help you learn about the brain. The site contains over three hundred color brain SPECT images, hundreds of scientific abstracts on brain SPECT imaging for psychiatry, a brain puzzle, and much, much more.

The SPECT color images relate to

aggression
attention deficit disorder, including the six subtypes
dementia and cognitive decline
drug abuse
PMS
anxiety disorders
brain trauma
depression
obsessive-compulsive disorder
stroke
seizures

Product Sources

Fish Oil Supplements

Coromega is made by European Reference Botanical Laboratories (ERBL); see www.coromega.com for information.

Nature's Mighty Bites, an incredible-tasting, healthy ice cream, contains high doses of omega-3 fatty acids; see www.kidsneedusnow.org for information.

For Nordic Naturals, Pro EPA, see www.nordicnaturals.com for information.

Other Treatment Resources

Red Rice Yeast Extract—cholesterol-lowering dietary supplement, red rice yeast extract can be purchased through Lifelink Nutritional Supplements at www.lifelinknet.com (see Chapter 6, page 154).

Low-Pressure Shunts—for information about the ongoing studies being performed by Eunoe, Inc., on low-pressure shunts for dementia, contact info@eunoe-inc.com or (888) 4MY-MIND or (888) 469-6463.

Acknowledgments

We are grateful to the best teachers that physicians can have—our patients. We wish to acknowledge and thank the staff of the Amen Clinics. We wish to thank Amanita Rosenbush (bookdok@earthlink.net) for editing consultation and help in blending our two sometimes very different styles of writing; Dr. Amen's research assistant, Lisa Rudy, who spent many hours helping us research the book, and whose brain drawings appear in the book; and Marian Kim and Angela Waldron, physician assistants at Amen Clinics, who helped gather the many images for the book. Thanks to Lucretia Reed, David Bennett, Kathleen Shores, Steve Rudolph, Sara Gilman, Dorothy Landing, and Ismael Mena, who read the manuscript and offered invaluable feedback.

Special thanks to Dr. Junko Hara (Dr. Shankle's amazing wife), who spent many hours encouraging us, reading the manuscript, and feeding us incredible food to get through the collaborative writing process. Her expertise in artificial intelligence, electrical engineering, business, human resource management, and Japanese society has allowed MCC to create a truly international service.

We would like to express our gratitude to Dr. Shankle's office assistant, Marisol Alvarado, whose hard work and compassion to ADRD patients and their families has greatly improved their lives; to Medial Care Corporation's (MCC) technical team, James Chen, Timothy Chan and Shannon Sun—who have pioneered new approaches to healthcare delivery; to Dennis Fortier, CEO of MCC, for his tireless commitment to bringing MCC's technology to the public and to healthcare professionals, and to MCC's and Shankle Clinic's supporters—Kenneth P. Simonds, Jason Paransky, Sharon Dugan, Martin McBirney, Dr. Anthony Clark and Dr. Sam Ho—who have worked to make a significant improvement in the lives of persons and their loved ones affected by Alzheimer's disease.

Posthumous thanks to Dr. Benjamin H. Landing, the oak tree from which the young acorn developed. Without him, Dr. Shankle would never have become a physician, and MCC would not exist. Also a special thanks to his wife and Dr. Shankle's mother, Dottie Landing, who passed on several genes of persistence to her son.

We are grateful to have a wonderful literary team. Our literary agent, Faith Hamlin, is one of the world's best agents. She remains a constant source of wisdom, love, and encouragement. Thanks also to our patient, thoughtful editor at Putnam, Sheila Curry Oakes.

Index

William Rodman Shankle, M.S., M.D.

Educated at Stanford University, Brown University, Harvard School of Public Health, and the University of Southern California and trained in medicine and neurology at Cook County and at LA County Hospitals, William Rodman Shankle is a neurologist and statistician who has diagnosed, treated, and managed over 7,000 patients and their families affected by Alzheimer's disease and related disorders (ADRD). He has devoted his entire career to researching how the brain functions during development, normal aging, and disease, and he has applied this knowledge to help people delay ADRD, preserve their independence, stay out of nursing homes, and lessen the burden on their loved ones.

In 1988, Dr. Shankle helped establish the Alzheimer's Disease Research Center at the University of California, Irvine, and he served as its medical director for ten years. During this time, the center became a member of the State of California Alzheimer's Disease Diagnosis and Treatment Centers and a member of the National Institute of Aging's Consortium to Establish a Registry for Alzheimer's Disease (CERAD).

In 1997, he started a community-based ADRD program to provide state-of-the-art healthcare to a larger public. He has also served as an advisor to the Japanese healthcare system in developing ADRD-based programs.

On January 4, 2000, *The New York Times* credited Dr. Shankle with having made one of the most important scientific discoveries and contributions of the 1990s—that the human brain doubles its number of neurons after birth. This discovery ushered in a new era of treatment for neurological disorders that uses the brain's own growth factors to generate stem cells that transform into nerve cells to replace dying ones.

Dr. Shankle recently received the prestigious Zenith Award from the Alzheimer's Association to develop affordable ways to detect ADRD before symptoms appear. He and his team have already developed automated screening (available at www.PreventAD.com) that can accurately detect ADRD up to eight years before it is currently diagnosed. The Society for Neuroscience recently recognized these efforts in a press release at their annual conference. Dr. Shankle has worked with Mrs. Maureen Reagan to help publicly promote the application of advanced technology to improve ADRD healthcare. He lectures throughout the United States and internationally and has made numerous appearances on television and radio. He has published more than fifty scientific, peer-reviewed studies.

Daniel G. Amen, M.D.

A clinical neuroscientist, psychiatrist, and the director of the Amen Clinics in Newport Beach and Fairfield, California, Tacoma, Washington, and Reston, Virginia, Daniel G. Amen, M.D., is a nationally recognized expert in the field of the brain and behavior, lecturing to thousands of psychiatrists, neurologists, psychologists, psychotherapists, and judges each year. Dr.

Amen has pioneered the clinical use of brain SPECT imaging in psychiatry. His clinics have the largest database in the world of brain images relating to behavior. He has presented his groundbreaking research on brain imaging and behavior internationally.

Dr. Amen did his psychiatric training at the Walter Reed Army Medical Center in Washington, D.C. He has won writing and research awards from the American Psychiatric Association, the United States Army, and the Baltimore-D.C. Institute for Psychoanalysis. Dr. Amen has been published around the world. He is the author of numerous professional and popular articles, nineteen books, and a number of audio and video programs. His books have been translated into over twelve languages and include *Change Your Brain, Change Your Life* (a *New York Times* bestseller), *Healing ADD, Healing the Hardware of the Soul,* and *Healing Anxiety and Depression.*